Integrative Medicine, Part I: Incorporating Complementary/Alternative Modalities

Guest Editor

J. ADAM RINDFLEISCH, MD, MPhil

PRIMARY CARE: CLINICS IN OFFICE PRACTICE

www.primarycare.theclinics.com

Consulting Editor
JOEL J. HEIDELBAUGH, MD

March 2010 • Volume 37 • Number 1

SAUNDERS an imprint of ELSEVIER, Inc.

W.B. SAUNDERS COMPANY
A Division of Elsevier Inc.

1600 John F. Kennedy Boulevard, Suite 1800 ● Philadelphia, PA 19103-2899

http://www.theclinics.com

PRIMARY CARE: CLINICS IN OFFICE PRACTICE Volume 37, Number 1
March 2010 ISSN 0095-4543, ISBN-13: 978-1-4377-1865-2

Editor: Barbara Cohen-Kligerman

Primary Care: Clinics in Office Practice (ISSN: 0095–4543) is published quarterly by Elsevier Inc., 360 Park Avenue South, New York, NY 10010-1710. Months of issue are March, June, September, and December. Periodicals postage paid at New York, NY and additional mailing offices. Subscription prices are $190.00 per year (US individuals), $320.00 (US institutions), $96.00 (US students), $232.00 (Canadian individuals), $376.00 (Canadian institutions), $151.00 (Canadian students), $289.00 (international individuals), $376.00 (international institutions), and $151.00 (international students). Foreign air speed delivery is included in all *Clinics* subscription prices. All prices are subject to change without notice. POSTMASTER: Send address changes to *Primary Care: Clinics in Office Practice*, Elsevier Periodicals Customer Service, 11830 Westline Industrial Drive, St. Louis, MO 63146. Customer Service Health Sciences Division, Subscription Customer Service, 3251 Riverport Lane, Maryland Heights, MO 63043. **Customer Service: 1-800-654-2452 (U.S. and Canada); 314-447-8871 (outside U.S. and Canada). Fax: 314-447-8029. E-mail: journalscustomerservice-usa@elsevier.com (for print support); journalsonlinesupport-usa@elsevier.com (for online support).**

Reprints. For copies of 100 or more, of articles in this publication, please contact the Commercial Reprints Department, Elsevier Inc., 360 Park Avenue South, New York, NY 10010-1710. Tel. (212) 633-3812; Fax: (212) 482-1935; E-mail: reprints@elsevier.com.

Primary Care: Clinics in Office Practice is covered in *MEDLINE/PubMed (Index Medicus)* and *EMBASE/ Excerpta Medica, Current Contents/Clinical Medicine,* and *ISI/BIOMED.*

Printed and bound by CPI Group (UK) Ltd, Croydon, CR0 4YY

Transferred to Digital Print 2011

Contributors

CONSULTING EDITOR

JOEL J. HEIDELBAUGH, MD
Clinical Assistant Professor and Clerkship Director, Department of Family Medicine;
Clinical Assistant Professor, Department of Urology, University of Michigan Medical
School, Ann Arbor, Michigan

GUEST EDITOR

J. ADAM RINDFLEISCH, MD, MPhil
Assistant Professor, Department of Family Medicine, University of Wisconsin School
of Medicine and Public Health, Odana Atrium Family Medicine Clinic, Madison, Wisconsin

AUTHORS

SAM CHASE, MFA, E-RYT
Sam Chase Yoga, Brooklyn, New York

BRIAN E. EARLEY, DO
Assistant Professor of Family Medicine (Clinical Health Sciences), University of Wisconsin
School of Medicine and Public Health, Madison, Wisconsin

SARA A. FLEMING, ND
Postdoctoral Research Fellow, Department of Family Medicine, University
of Wisconsin-Madison, Madison, Wisconsin

LUKE FORTNEY, MD
Assistant Professor, Department of Family Medicine, University of Wisconsin-Madison;
UW Health Odana Atrium Family Medicine Clinic, Madison, Wisconsin

NEELIMA GANTA, MD
Family Medicine Resident, Central Maine Medical Center Family Medicine Residency,
Lewiston, Maine

RONALD M. GLICK, MD
Assistant Professor of Psychiatry, Physical Medicine and Rehabilitation, and Family
Medicine, University of Pittsburgh School of Medicine; Medical Director, Center for
Integrative Medicine at UPMC Shadyside, Pittsburgh, Pennsylvania

CAROL M. GRECO, PhD
Assistant Professor of Psychiatry, University of Pittsburgh School of Medicine, Center for
Integrative Medicine at UPMC Shadyside, Pittsburgh, Pennsylvania

NANCY C. GUTKNECHT, ND
Postdoctoral Research Fellow, Department of Family Medicine, University of Wisconsin-Madison, Madison, Wisconsin

MARSHA J. HANDEL, MLS
Director, Informatics and Online Education, Department of Integrative Medicine, Beth Israel Medical Center, New York, New York

MEG HAYES, MD
Associate Professor, Oregon Health & Science University, Portland, Oregon

MICHAEL T. HERNKE, PhD
Research Fellow, Lecturer, Department of Operations & Information Management, School of Business, University of Wisconsin-Madison, Madison, Wisconsin

RAHUL KAPUR, MD, CAQSM
Assistant Director, Primary Care Sports Medicine Fellowship; Assistant Professor, Family Medicine and Sports Medicine, Department of Family Medicine and Community Health, University of Pennsylvania Sports Medicine Center, University of Pennsylvania Health System, Philadelphia, Pennsylvania

ERICA LOVETT, MD
Integrative Family Medicine Physician and Faculty, Central Maine Medical Center Family Medicine Residency, Lewiston, Maine

HELEN LUCE, DO
Assistant Professor of Family Medicine (Clinical Health Sciences), University of Wisconsin School of Medicine and Public Health, Wausau, Wisconsin

JILL MALLORY, MD
Fellow, Academic Integrative Medicine, Department of Family Medicine, Odana Atrium Family Medicine Clinic; Clinical Instructor, Department of Family Medicine, School of Medicine and Public Health, University of Wisconsin, Madison, Wisconsin

JUN J. MAO, MD, MSCE
Assistant Professor and Director of Integrative Medicine, Department of Family Medicine and Community Health, University of Pennsylvania, Philadelphia, Pennsylvania

RIAN J. PODEIN, MD
Assistant Professor, Department of Family Medicine, University of Wisconsin School of Medicine and Public Health, Madison, Wisconsin

DAVID RABAGO, MD
Department of Family Medicine, University of Wisconsin School of Medicine and Public Health, Madison, Wisconsin

DAVE RAKEL, MD
Associate Professor, Department of Family Medicine, Odana Atrium Family Medicine Clinic, University of Wisconsin, Madison, Wisconsin; UW Health Integrative Medicine Director

J. ADAM RINDFLEISCH, MD, MPhil
Assistant Professor, Department of Family Medicine, University of Wisconsin School of Medicine and Public Health, Odana Atrium Family Medicine Clinic, Madison, Wisconsin

ANDREW SLATTENGREN, DO
Department of Family Medicine, University of Wisconsin School of Medicine and Public Health, Madison, Wisconsin

MOLLY TAYLOR, BS
Second Year Medical Student, Dartmouth Medical School, Hanover, New Hampshire

ALEKSANDRA ZGIERSKA, MD, PhD
Department of Family Medicine, University of Wisconsin School of Medicine and Public Health, Madison, Wisconsin

Contents

> Integrative medicine is healing-oriented medicine that accounts for the whole person (body, mind, and spirit), including all aspects of lifestyle. Integrative medicine emphasizes the therapeutic relationship and makes use of all appropriate therapies, both conventional and alternative. This article describes ways to bring the integrative perspective into primary care practice. Several approaches are described, including some that are routinely used in the authors' practice. Changes in practice philosophy that can (1) help inform primary care redesign, (2) facilitate the creation of patient-centered medical homes, (3) strengthen provider-patient relationships, and (4) enhance patient satisfaction are also provided.

> Herbs and nutraceuticals are commonly used in many households in the United States. This article discusses supplement use patterns and offers resources for primary care providers wishing to counsel patients more effectively about dietary supplements. Supplement safety issues, types of herbal formulations, and a summary of the uses, doses, side effects, and evidence ratings for 10 commonly used herbs and 11 commonly used nutraceuticals are provided.

> More than 15.8 million people in the United States now practice some form of yoga, and nearly half of current practitioners stated they began yoga practice as a means of improving overall health. More broadly understood in a modern context, yoga is a set of principles and practices designed to promote health and well-being through the integration of body, breath, and mind. This article outlines the history of yoga and describes several forms, including asana-based yoga, which is becoming popular in the United States. Research findings related to use of yoga as a therapy for various health problems are reviewed. Guidelines for finding a yoga teacher are offered, as are a number of book and Internet sources of further information.

processes. Successful treatment employing biofeedback can be beneficial for several stress-related and pain conditions, as well as other forms
of somatic disturbance. Collectively, the same conditions that may respond to biofeedback are those often seen in a primary care practice
and are conditions that can result in chronic dysfunction and disability. Understanding the forms and uses of biofeedback, the research evidence
base, and practical referral guidelines can help the family physician to offer
recommendations and referrals to patients.

Acupuncture, an ancient traditional Chinese medical therapy, is used
widely around the world. When practiced by a certified provider, it is
safe and patients often find it calming and relaxing. Animal and human
studies have found a physiologic basis for acupuncture needling in that
it affects the complex central and peripheral neurohormonal network. Although it is unclear whether acupuncture is beneficial over sham/placebo
acupuncture, acupuncture care yields clinically relevant short- and long-
term benefits for low back pain, knee osteoarthritis, chronic neck pain,
and headache. The integration of acupuncture into a primary care setting
also appears to be cost-effective. The practice of acupuncture in primary
care requires rigorous training, financial discipline, and good communication skills. When done correctly, acupuncture is beneficial for both patients
and providers.

Naturopathy is a distinct type of primary care medicine that blends age-old
healing traditions with scientific advances and current research. Naturopathy is guided by a unique set of principles that recognize the body's innate healing capacity, emphasize disease prevention, and encourage
individual responsibility to obtain optimal health. Naturopathic treatment
modalities include diet and clinical nutrition, behavioral change, hydrotherapy, homeopathy, botanical medicine, physical medicine, pharmaceuticals, and minor surgery. Naturopathic physicians (NDs) are trained as
primary care physicians in 4-year, accredited doctoral-level naturopathic
medical schools. At present, there are 15 US states, 2 US territories,
and several provinces in Canada, Australia, and New Zealand that recognize licensure for NDs.

Unsustainable development around the world has contributed to ecological degradation and human suffering while compromising the ability of
ecosystems and social institutions to support human life. The United
States health care system and its institutions are significant contributors
to unsustainable development, but leaders of change are emerging from
the health care arena. Health professionals, including primary care

providers, are poised to serve as models for sustainability and to facilitate the necessary transformation toward more sustainable practices. Health professionals must, within a practical framework, embrace an objective definition of sustainability and then act to achieve it.

Jill Mallory

There are many options for natural and preventative therapies during pregnancy and childbirth, which may aid in minimizing the use of pharmaceuticals and invasive procedures. Patients may seek these out, and it is important for physicians to have some basic knowledge to guide their choices. Of all therapies, the most important are nutrition for optimizing health and the provision of continuous support during labor.

J. Adam Rindfleisch

Energy medicine modalities, also known as biofield therapies, are perhaps the most mysterious and controversial complementary alternative medicine therapies. Although many of these approaches have existed for millennia, scientific investigation of these techniques is in its early stages; much remains to be learned about mechanisms of action and efficacy. These techniques are increasingly used in clinical and hospital settings and can be incorporated into an integrative primary care practice. This article describes several energy medicine and biofield therapies and outlines key elements they hold in common. Several specific approaches are described. Research findings related to the efficacy of energy medicine are summarized, and proposed mechanisms of action and safety issues are discussed. Guidelines are offered for primary care providers wishing to advise patients about energy medicine or to integrate it into their practices, and Internet and other resources for obtaining additional information are provided.

Marsha J. Handel

The Internet: gateway to reliable clinical and research information or floodgate to unsubstantiated information of insufficient depth and variable quality? Can it help the physician locate high-quality information that will enhance patient care? Can it help patients become more knowledgeable, involved, and competent in participating in their health care management? Can it be used efficiently and effectively during a busy practice day to immediately educate providers and patients right at point of care? The answer to all these questions is yes. This article will empower readers with knowledge of authoritative Web sites that directly addresses clinical questions, are easy to search, and will help physicians guide their patients to sources of information that are valid and trustworthy.

VISIT THE CLINICS ONLINE!

Access your subscription at:
www.theclinics.com

Foreword
Traditional Medicine in Primary Care is Not Enough: We Must All Integrate CAM!

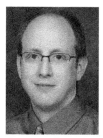

Joel J. Heidelbaugh, MD
Consulting Editor

It's inescapable: Complementary and alternative medicine (CAM) is not only here to stay, but it also continues to permeate our lives in popularity, prevalence, and necessity. Moreover, clinical and translational research in this arena has proven that a myriad of nonconventional therapies provide benefit for many disorders that ail us, and waves of outcomes-based data continue to demonstrate impressive efficacy. From herbs to nutritional supplements, meditation to yoga, biofeedback to acupuncture, these and other modalities have piqued our interest and improved the lives of many of us and of people we know. In our daily routine of conventional medical practice, we must ask ourselves: "Is what we're doing for our patients adequate enough?" "What other resources can I use to help my patients achieve their goals and minimize their risk of morbidity and mortality?" Ultimately: "Could integrating CAM practices enable us to offer better education to our patients regarding healthier lifestyle choices and disease prevention?"

The "necessity" component of CAM in our society should not go overlooked. Centered on the biopsychosocial approach to patient care, it enables us to create the ideal paradigm on which primary care is centered: namely, taking care of the "whole patient." The various components of CAM bring great optimism toward the management of chronic diseases, including cardiac, gastrointestinal, endocrinologic, pulmonary, and rheumatologic conditions, as well as the potential for managing many others. We can only hope that the future of health care turns more attention toward offering CAM services as an integral part of primary care, and that these services will become covered benefits by insurance payers.

Clinicians stand to learn a great deal from current and advancing CAM practices. Unfortunately, the great majority of this learning must occur after completion of

Prim Care Clin Office Pract 37 (2010) xiii–xiv
doi:10.1016/j.pop.2009.11.001   primarycare.theclinics.com

medical school and residency, as only a few clinicians pursue additional specialized training and even fewer feel comfortable incorporating such knowledge in their practices. According to the American Association of Medical Colleges, 113 of 126 medical schools in 2008 required courses in CAM, while 77 schools offered elective courses in this discipline. However, among schools that required such courses, only 4.4 hours in the preclinical years and 3.1 hours in the clinical clerkships were dedicated to CAM.[1] Despite this exposure, we continue to produce clinicians who have insufficient understanding and skill in integrating CAM modalities in their daily practices. Similarly, most clinicians are not equipped to answer their patients' questions regarding even the most basic principles of integrative medicine.

As the consulting editor for *Primary Care Clinics*, the consistent advice I give to guest editors is to work closely with their authors to create a novel publication that contains current and salient evidence-based practice guidelines highlighting what they would need to enhance their everyday practices and enrich their teaching experiences. Dr Adam Rindfleisch has mastered this assignment, coupling his extensive background of clinical practice and research experience in CAM with that of his authors, to deliver a unique and informative issue that serves as the first of two issues dedicated to this topic. Readers will discover and enjoy well-crafted literature reviews featuring principles of osteopathic medicine, naturopathy and nutraceuticals, meditation and biofeedback, yoga, and acupuncture. Quite impressive is a review that discusses integrating sustainability in health care. This source, providing vast amounts of information for clinicians across all fields of medicine, enables readers to easily integrate this new knowledge into their practices and to enrich their own lives.

Joel J. Heidelbaugh, MD
Departments of Family Medicine and Urology
University of Michigan Medical School
Ann Arbor, MI, USA
and
Ypsilanti Health Center
200 Arnet Street, Suite 200
Ypsilanti, MI 48198, USA

E-mail address:
jheidel@umich.edu

REFERENCE

1. Association of American Medical Colleges. US medical schools teaching selected topics 2008 LCME part II annual medical school questionnaire. Retrieved from the World Wide Web on October 25, 2009. Available at: http://services.aamc.org/currdir/section2/2008hottopics.pdf. Accessed October 25, 2009.

Preface
Integrative Medicine in Primary Care

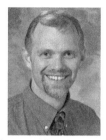

J. Adam Rindfleisch, MD, MPhil
Guest Editor

In recent years, we have been hearing about—and directly experiencing—many trends that affect primary care. Primary care providers are in short supply.[1] We do a great deal of uncompensated work.[2] Some say we are the key to "fixing" the broken US health care system.[3] We are encouraged to build medical homes,[4] recruit more students into primary care,[3] and adopt new technologies, such as electronic medical records.[5] Meanwhile, primary care providers continue to confront the never-ending daily challenge of seeing as many patients as possible without compromising the quality of care we provide or the balance between our professional and personal lives. It is no surprise that we are said to be at high risk for burnout,[6] with many of us transitioning to hospitalist medicine, intermediate care, or other pursuits.[7]

For all the challenges we face, however, there is reason for optimism. Ample opportunity exists, in the context of all these shifts, to reinvent our profession, exploring new ways to meet patients' needs, enrich our practices, and reconnect with the reasons we became primary care providers in the first place.

This issue's main objective is to explore how integrative medicine (IM) might inform primary care. Defined in detail in the first article of this volume, IM draws from complementary and alternative medicine, with an emphasis on evidence-based practice and safety. Beyond that, IM is an overall philosophy of care; it is primary care par excellence, emphasizing provider-patient relationships, the innate human capacity for healing, individualization of care, and use of a holistic (bio-psycho-social-spiritual) approach. IM focuses on prevention, healthy lifestyle choices, and fresh approaches to chronic disease management. It also promotes provider self-care, an all-too-often ignored aspect of our work.

Patients want this approach. In 2007, according to the National Health Interview Survey, 4 out of 10 adults and 1 out of 9 children were reported to use some form of complementary and alternative medicine.[8] Over $38 million was spent on 354.2 million

Prim Care Clin Office Pract 37 (2010) xv–xvii
doi:10.1016/j.pop.2009.09.014
0095-4543/10/$ – see front matter © 2010 Elsevier Inc. All rights reserved.

primarycare.theclinics.com

visits, most of which was paid out of pocket.[9] People state they use these services because they are safer, more individualized, less invasive, and more consistent with their beliefs about their health.

As my practice partners and I have worked to create an integrative primary care model over the past few years, we have found the process fulfilling and frustrating at times. Challenges have included resistance from some colleagues (though most of them are quite supportive of IM), outdated reimbursement structures, and simply not having enough time to incorporate new ideas. Positives have included enhanced patient satisfaction, having more to offer patients (in particular those with chronic conditions), and seeing burgeoning interest in IM among the medical students and residents we teach.

I do not pretend that merging IM with primary care is a panacea that will heal all of primary care's woes, but it does have a great deal to offer, as recently highlighted at an Institute of Medicine summit on IM.[10] The articles in this issue offer many resources for primary care providers to consider using if they find themselves drawn to the integrative model of care. To successfully meet current challenges, we must explore new ways to practice, guided by an unflagging commitment to bring optimal health to patients and providers alike.

A variety of treatment modalities are discussed in these articles, and many of them pose certain challenges to those who wish to study them - or interpret study findings. Not all complementary and alternative modalities can easily be studied in randomized controlled trials; in many instances, defining control groups, gauging what constitutes a significant treatment effect, and even offering a given modality's mechanism of action have been topics of heated debate. I commend the authors of this volume for investing a great deal of effort into rating research findings. Key points given an A rating have been deemed by the author to have consistent and good-quality, patient-oriented evidence supporting them. B ratings are given when patient-oriented evidence is available but limited or inconsistent, and C ratings are given when support comes from other sources such as consensus, usual practice, or opinion without a strong evidence base. These ratings are, at some level, subject to interpretation.

My sincere thanks to all those affiliated with University of Wisconsin Integrative Medicine, trailblazers all, and specifically to my practice partners, who make exploring the frontiers of medicine an adventure. Special thanks to my family for their patience as I undertook this project and to Barbara Cohen-Kligerman and Dr Joel Heidelbaugh for all of their guidance. Thank you to my patients, many of whom have been my greatest teachers. Finally, my gratitude to all the authors without whose creativity and expertise this publication would not have been possible. In these turbulent times, it is heartening to witness the commitment and dedication so many people feel about the preservation—and evolution—of primary care.

J. Adam Rindfleisch, MD, MPhil
Department of Family Medicine, University of Wisconsin School of Medicine and
Public Health
Odana Atrium Family Medicine Clinic
5618 Odana Road
Madison, WI 53719, USA

E-mail address:
adam.rindfleisch@fammed.wisc.edu

REFERENCES

1. Cross M. What the primary care physician shortage means for managed health plans. Manag Care 2009; Available at: http://www.managedcaremag.com/archives/0706/0706.shortage.html. Accessed August 31, 2009.
2. Biola H, Green LA, Phillips RL, Guirguis-Blake J, et al. The US primary care physician workforce: undervalued service. Am Fam Physician 2003;68(8):1486.
3. Wang S.S. Obama: 'severe shortage' of primary care docs. Wall Street Journal Health Blog. Available at: http://blogs.wsj.com/health/2009/08/11/obama-primary-care-docs-make-a-lot–less-money-than-specialists/. Accessed August 31, 2009.
4. Patient-centered primary care collaborative website. Available at: http://www.pcpcc.net/. Accessed August 31, 2009.
5. Goldner D. Obama's big idea: digital health records. CNN money.com. Available at: http://money.cnn.com/2009/01/12/technology/stimulus_health_care/. Accessed August 31, 2009. Available at: http://www.cnn.com/2009/HEALTH/08/25/harris.primary.care.doctor/index.html. Accessed August 31, 2009.
6. Anderson S, Gabbe SG, Christensen JF. Mid-career burnout in generalist and specialist physicians. JAMA 2002;288:1447–50.
7. Harris V. Commentary: why primary care doctors are fed up. Available at: http://www.cnn.com/2009/HEALTH/08/25/harris.primary.care.doctor/index.html. Accessed August 31, 2009.
8. Barnes PM, Bloom B. Complementary and alternative medicine use among adults and children: United States, 2007. Natl Health Stat Report, 2008; 12. Available at: http://nccam.nih.gov/news/2008/nhsr12.pdf. Accessed August 20, 2009.
9. Nahin RL, Barnes PM, Stassman BJ, Bloom B. Costs of complementary and alternative medicine (CAM) and frequency of visits to CAM practitioners: United States, 2007. Natl Health Stat Report 2009;18.
10. National Institute of Medicine, 2009 Summit on integrative medicine and the health of the public. Available at: http://www.iom.edu/?ID=52555. Accessed August 31, 2009.

Introduction to Integrative Primary Care: The Health-Oriented Clinic

Luke Fortney, MD[a],*, Dave Rakel, MD[a],
J. Adam Rindfleisch, MD, MPhil[a], Jill Mallory, MD[b]

KEYWORDS

• Integrative medicine • Primary care • Prevention • Wellness

DEFINING INTEGRATIVE MEDICINE

Integrative medicine (IM) is healing-oriented medicine that takes account of the whole person (body, mind, and spirit), including all aspects of lifestyle. IM emphasizes the therapeutic relationship and makes use of all appropriate therapies, both conventional and alternative.[19] The term "integrative medicine" was coined in the 1990s to encourage the integration of complementary and alternative medicine (CAM) with conventional therapies to facilitate health and disease prevention. At that time, basic foundational ingredients of well-being, such as nutrition, the mind-body connection, and spirituality, were defined as CAM.[20] It has become increasingly obvious that it is difficult to define health without these basic components. As the culture of medicine evolves, IM becomes less concerned about labeling various therapies as CAM, focusing instead on developing insight into therapies that are needed to create optimal health. Making health the primary objective allows the professionals in the CAM and allopathic communities to collaborate to establish excellence in health creation (salutogenesis) for the communities they serve (**Box 1**).

In 2009, the Institute of Medicine (IOM) sponsored a Summit on Integrative Medicine and the Health of the Public. IOM President Harvey Fineberg described common themes that professionals from diverse disciplines can use to create new models of health-oriented care:

[a] Department of Family Medicine, Odana Atrium Family Medicine Clinic, University of Wisconsin, 5618 Odana Road, Madison, WI 53719, USA
[b] Academic Integrative Medicine, Department of Family Medicine, Odana Atrium Family Medicine Clinic, University of Wisconsin, 5618 Odana Road, Madison, WI 53719, USA
* Corresponding author.
E-mail address: luke.fortney@fammed.wisc.edu (L. Fortney).

Prim Care Clin Office Pract 37 (2010) 1–12
doi:10.1016/j.pop.2009.09.003
0095-4543/10/$ – see front matter. Published by Elsevier Inc.
primarycare.theclinics.com

Key Points	Evidence Rating	Reference(s)
Salutogenesis-oriented sessions have the potential to improve patient satisfaction and outcomes	C	1
Health-oriented teams have the potential to enhance the quality of health care	C	1,2
Strong therapeutic partnerships enhance the quality of primary care and decrease care costs	B	3–5
Effective communication enhances care	B	6,7
Matching explanations of care to a patient's value system enhances care	B	8,9
Support and follow-up improve care	B	1,2
More time with providers improves patient satisfaction	B	10
Healthy behaviors of providers foster healthy behaviors and lifestyle changes in patients	A	11,12
Inquiring about healthy behaviors increases likelihood that they will change	B	13,14
Empathy and compassion enhance care	A	15
The personality of a provider is a determinant of treatment response	B	16
Home visits improve quality of care	B	17
Education in integrative medicine makes it more acceptable in various practice environments	B	18

1. An understanding that health is more important than the absence of disease
2. A recognition that health is influenced not only by physical or genetic factors but also by emotional, psychosocial, environmental, and spiritual aspects
3. A focus on health maintenance and disease prevention as well as acute and chronic care
4. An emphasis on interdisciplinary collaboration
5. Acknowledgment of biologic variation and the need to treat individuals, not statistical averages.[21]

It is important to acknowledge that health-oriented medicine takes into account and supports the health and wellness of the clinician, with the understanding that one cannot give what one does not have.

INTEGRATIVE MEDICINE IN PRIMARY CARE: KEY INGREDIENTS

Primary care is the most appropriate venue for IM. Primary care allows for continuous relationships that lead to an understanding of barriers of self-healing. Behaviors such as healthy eating, regular physical activity, and avoiding toxic substances are the main

---

Box 1
Principles of integrative medicine

- Patient and practitioner are partners in the healing process.
- All factors that influence health, wellness, and disease, including mind, spirit, community, and body, are taken into consideration.
- Appropriate use of conventional and alternative methods facilitates the body's innate healing response.
- Effective interventions that are natural and less invasive should be used whenever possible.
- Good medicine is based on good science. It is inquiry driven and open to new paradigms.
- Ultimately, the patient must decide how to proceed with treatment based on values, beliefs, and available evidence.
- Along with the concept of treatment, the broader concepts of health promotion and the prevention of illness are also paramount.
- Practitioners of integrative medicine (IM) should exemplify its principles and commit themselves to self-exploration and self-development, understanding that practitioners "cannot give what they do not have."
- Rather than being its own specialty area, IM is an overall approach and framework that can be incorporated into all branches of allopathic medicine.

From Maizes V, Rakel D, Niemiec C. Integrative medicine and patient-centered care. 2009:35. Available at: http://www.iom.edu/Object.File/Master/62/372/Integrative%20Medicine%20and %20Patient%20Centered%20Care.pdf. Accessed June 27, 2009.

---

driving forces for reducing morbidity and mortality.[22] Emotional influences often shape these behaviors, and they can be influenced most positively through relationships with family members, friends, and members of the primary care team. As primary care redefines itself through the patient-centered medical home model, there is an opportunity for the health-oriented clinic to act as a seamless transition between the polarities of health and disease, moving toward the former.[23] This transition requires a shift in intention toward health as a valued outcome.

SALUTOGENESIS-ORIENTED SESSION

In primary care, to focus more on health it is essential to create office visits that have health and healing as their primary goal. The term "salutogenesis", which means "the creation of health," was introduced by the American-Israeli medical sociologist Aaron Antonovsky,[24] who was interested in exploring the origin of health than in looking for the cause of disease (pathogenesis). The investment in developing a relationship over time creates a "context of understanding" in which unique wellness needs of the individual are discovered and supported. With gentle and directed questioning, patients often self-discover and disclose the root cause of their symptoms, and see for themselves what is needed for their resolution. If providers do not have time to listen, the patient often becomes a passive recipient of treatments rather than an active participant in the healing process (**Table 1**).

HEALTH-ORIENTED TEAMS

The salutogenesis-oriented session (SOS) often requires collaboration with other professionals who are best suited to help guide the patient toward health in different ways.

Table 1
Key practitioner influences for a successful salutogenesis-oriented session

Practitioner Goals	Reasoning/Evidence
1. Develop a trusting relationship	It is through relationship that the patient feels comfortable expressing emotions, resulting in optimism and positive expectation[3,4]
2. Listen with intent and empathy to the patient's story	Being fully present with positive intention is perceived positively by patients and enhances the healing effects of the encounter.[25] It is important that the patient feels understood
3. Provide an explanation for the patient's problem	The explanation makes sense of a chaotic and threatening situation resulting in an enhanced sense of control[26]
4. Match the explanation to the patient's culture, beliefs, and values	Matching the explanation to the patient's own values allows for the development of insight.[8] It puts the problem within a context that is accepted and creates buy-in[9]
5. The explanation is accepted by the patient, and it creates insight	Acceptance of the explanation leads to treatment and positive expectation. This results in healing, even if the explanation is not true.[27] The art of medicine is when we can reproduce this effect without deception
6. Create a plan that leads to action, empowerment, and positive expectation	If the above goals are successful, the patient will be more likely to engage in a plan that empowers her/him to make changes that result in more sustainable effects toward health[28,29]
7. Provide support and follow-up	Providing ongoing support and collaboration with other providers is the hallmark of primary care and supports a continuous healing relationship[1,2]

From Rakel D. The salutogenesis-oriented session: creating space and time for healing in primary care. Explore (NY) 2008;4:42–7; with permission.

A team of professionals working toward the creation of health is different from the one that is focused on treating disease. Ideally, the incorporation and integration of these teams will result in decreased need for disease-oriented teams such as those already in place to treat conditions such as renal failure, heart disease, and diabetes (**Table 2**).

The creation of health-oriented teams also allows for improved access to health services that is not limited by the bottleneck of a required physician visit (**Fig. 1**). For example, a person with depression can first see a psychologist to explore the origins of depression. The psychologist can then collaborate with the primary care clinician if more aggressive therapy is needed. Similarly, people with abnormal lipids can see a nutritionist first and then if laboratory goals are not met, can follow up with the primary care clinician for pharmaceutical therapy. The shortage of primary care clinicians[30] demands a team-oriented approach that honors how health professionals can work together toward a common goal. This approach will improve care while reducing suffering and the high costs of treating diseases late in their progression.

THERAPEUTIC PARTNERSHIP AND THE HEALTH AGREEMENT

The therapeutic relationship is the cornerstone of integrative primary care in which patient and practitioner are partners in the healing process. Including patients as active participants in their own medical decision making is an empowering and effective way to facilitate healing. Relationship-centered care allows practitioner and patient to communicate more effectively to get to the root of the patient's concern.

Table 2
The health-oriented team

Health Ingredient	Health Professional (Examples)
Nutrition	Nutritionist, registered dietician
Exercise and movement	Exercise physiologist, yoga instructor, health coach
Emotional health	Psychologist, licensed social worker, mindfulness teacher
Spiritual connection	Chaplain, spiritual guide, pastor, rabbi, priest
Behavior change	Psychologist, social worker, health coach
Removing barriers	Social worker, case manager, health coach
Therapeutic touch	Osteopath, chiropractor, massage therapist, healing touch provider, reiki practitioner

Good communication comes from developing rapport and empathy with the patient, which in turn supports and informs diagnosis and treatment.

As the practitioner-patient relationship develops, significant health benefits ensue that have been found to improve efficiency of care by reducing dependence on excessive tests and referrals.[5] Compassionately asked, provocative, far-reaching questions about lifestyle and beliefs not only deepen the therapeutic relationship but also lead to new insights that help patients recognize for themselves which behaviors are consistent or inconsistent with their stated goals and values.[6,7] This aspect is particularly important because research suggests that psychosocial factors continue to be overlooked in the clinical setting.[31,32]

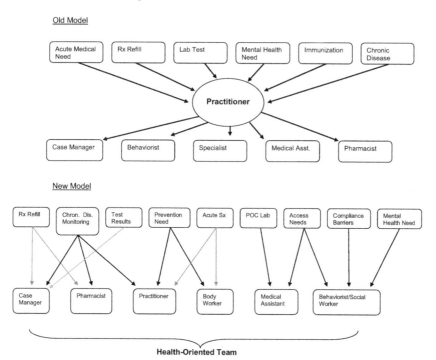

Fig. 1. Old and new models of health services. POC, point of care; Rx, prescription; Sx, symptoms. *From* Gottlieb K, Sylvester I, Eby D. Transforming your practice—what matters most. Fam Pract Manag 2008;15:32–8; with permission.

Authentically being present with the patient and listening to their concerns can help reveal undiscovered biologic, psychological, and social factors that affect his or her health. For the clinician, being mindfully present may influence the healing process and catalyze the patient's motivation for real change. This type of therapeutic interaction may require additional time per visit (SOS visits may take 40–60 minutes), but it is important to patients and has clinical value. For example, patient-satisfaction scores directly correlate with the amount of perceived time spent with the health practitioner.[10] In addition, how health practitioners are perceived by patients has direct effects on behavior and health outcomes. In a study by Rakel and colleagues,[15] patients with common cold who perceived their physician as being more empathetic showed significantly reduced severity and duration of cold symptoms. Another study found that one-third of psychiatrists treating patients with placebo were more effective in treating depression than another one-third of psychiatrists who were treating patients with imipramine, further emphasizing the point that therapeutic presence and practice style affect health outcomes.[16] **Box 2** shows examples of healing-oriented questions.

Health practitioners should exemplify the principles of wellness and commit themselves to self-care. The Healthy Doctor Healthy Patient Project shows that physicians who regularly engage themselves in physical activity are better at counseling their patients about exercise.[11] Physicians' disclosures of their own healthy behaviors improve credibility and ability to motivate the patient. This aspect is especially relevant because a major challenge of clinical practice is promoting behavior change, particularly when one considers that 40% of all mortality stems from unhealthy behaviors,

---

Box 2
Examples of healing-oriented questions

What do you believe is the root of these symptoms?

Asking "what do you believe" (vs "what do you think") allows for the patient to reflect on what they think is going on. Asking "what do you think" attaches a cognitive context of right versus wrong and removes the invitation to express emotions that may not have a right answer.

If this illness has created a hole within you, what do you fill this hole with?

Opportunity to explore what gives the patient a sense of meaning and purpose.

If anything were possible, what would your ideal life look like?

Inquire about potential barriers or ingredients that give meaning to life.

In a time of difficulty, whom do you turn to for support?

Explore social support and sense of community.

When these symptoms started, were there any stressful events happening in your life?

Brings awareness of how stressful life events can be internalized causing somatic symptoms.

You know yourself better than anyone. If you were your own doctor, how would you treat this condition?

Provides information on what the patient believes they need most. This should be incorporated into the health plan.

Listen for metaphor: You said that your job is "eating you up inside." Do you feel that this is related to your abdominal pain and heartburn?

Metaphor is an opportunity to bring insight into the importance of the mind-body influences on health.

such as smoking, alcohol use, overeating, sedentary lifestyle, and unsafe sexual practices.[12] In a study by Frank and colleagues,[33] patients counseled by a physician who revealed brief information about her own healthy dietary and exercise practices, and had a bike helmet and apple visible on her desk, considered her to be healthier, more believable, and more motivating than patients in a control group who did not receive this kind of disclosure.

Considering that brief advice from a physician leads to a spontaneous quit rate of 2% to 4%, just from asking about tobacco use, it is reasonable to infer that inquiring about other health behaviors would effect real change also.[13,14] One proposal involves formal reviewing of major areas of lifestyle that promote disease prevention and wellness with every annual physical examination. Offering brief suggestions based on personal and professional experience can help strengthen the therapeutic relationship between practitioner and patient, and improve clinical outcomes. Reviewing a formal "health agreement" with patients on a yearly basis is a practical example of a harmless way to be proactive with patient-centered care that incorporates health intent into the primary care setting.

It is also important to acknowledge that "you cannot give what you do not have." "Walking the talk" and embodying the health the practitioners encourage in their patients is an essential piece of integrative primary care. Every small step in the direction of personal and professional wellness translates into more authentic communication and relationship with the patients, which is the keystone of good medical care.

To optimize a wellness-oriented, relationship-centered approach, the authors devised a Health Agreement (**Box 3**), which is reviewed during every new patient visit, physical examination, or SOS.

HOME VISITS: THE EXAMPLE OF BREAST-FEEDING

Home visiting is a mutually satisfying part of an integrative practice model that can help strengthen the therapeutic relationship. Populations that may especially benefit include the handicapped, elderly, postpartum women, and newborns. In general, patients appreciate the personal attention and convenience of having their primary care practitioner visit their home, and care providers also feel they gain enormous insight into their patients' lives.[17]

One of the most important benefits of having a home visit program is the optimal support of breast-feeding.[34] It is well known that the first 2 weeks of a newborn baby's life is a critical time for maternal-infant bonding, for learning feeding techniques and hunger cues, and for establishing an optimal milk supply, which are important for the health of the infant and the mother. Because current societal trends of bottle-feeding often leave new mothers with an insecure feeling about breast-feeding, it is important that new mothers have strong support and guidance from their physicians.[35] The clinician can also observe the home environment to counsel the mother about how to deal with pressures, which might be separating her from her newborn during this critical period.

It is often said that the birth of a child is an opportunity for all who are involved to learn to become servants. Likewise, at the other end of the spectrum, end-of-life care and hospice home visits by the primary care practitioner can greatly improve the quality of patient care. These are precious times for families when the health practitioner can further serve the needs of the family. The clinician comes to the home to provide supportive care and to be an encouraging advisor at the bedside of the family. This visit is a unique opportunity for a mutually satisfying patient encounter, which reconnects the health provider with beauty and meaning in the practice of medicine.

Box 3
The Health Agreement

Welcome to our clinic. Our focus is your health, but to succeed we need your help. We may only spend a few hours together each year, setting the stage for how you can optimize health and well-being the rest of the time. While it is vital to keep all your parts working and to fix them when needed, we also want to focus on you as a *whole person*. This means paying attention to emotions, thoughts, beliefs, and relationships—all the things that make you who you are. If you do this, you will be sick less often, will need fewer drugs and procedures, and will have a better quality of life. Please join us in committing to your wellness.

I, _____ , will do my best to promote my own health. I acknowledge that the following areas are beneficial to my well-being:

1. *Movement and/or exercise.* I will try to do some form of vigorous movement or exercise most days of the week.

2. *A healthy diet.* I will try to eat at least 5 servings (*1 serving size ~ the size of the palm of your hand*) of fresh fruits and vegetables daily. When possible, I will use organic and locally produced food, including multicolored whole foods. I will try to limit foods that are processed or have many artificial ingredients.

3. *Rest.* I acknowledge that my body and mind need rest in order to heal and restore. I will try to get enough sleep each night, and I will take short naps during the day if needed.

4. *A healthy weight.* I will do my best to move toward and maintain a body type that is healthy for me.

5. *Avoiding harmful substances.* If there is a substance or habit that I use too much and would have trouble giving up, such as food, caffeine, tobacco, alcohol, drugs, anger, guilt, or low self-esteem, I will seek help in letting it go.

6. *Healthy relationships.* I will focus on having healthy family ties, friendships, sexual connections, and other types of relationships. I understand that caring for others and being cared for is good for me and my community.

7. *Managing stress.* I understand that the body and mind are connected. When one suffers, the other is also affected. I will mindfully pay attention to how I feel stress in my body and explore ways to ease this.

8. *Connecting with nature.* I acknowledge that the environment influences my health, and I will do my best to help protect it. Being in nature is healing and I will spend time exploring it.

9. *Spiritual connection.* Spirituality is something that I define for myself. I recognize that being helpful and kind to others is good for me. I will reflect on what gives my life meaning and purpose, and I will do my best to help it grow and share it with others.

10. *Maintaining balance.* I acknowledge that time for myself, with others, and for play is just as important as work and finances. I will do my best to find balance in my life.

I will do my best to practice these healthful habits. I feel I should start with number(s)_____

Health Partner: _____

As your health care practitioner, I will help you work toward these goals. I will do my best to be available and attentive to your needs in a way that assists your own capacity to heal.

Healthcare Practitioner: _____

EDUCATION: TRAINING IN PRIMARY CARE INTEGRATIVE MEDICINE

Education is a vital piece in the creation of an integrative primary care practice. Many providers, particularly those who have been in practice for some time, have received little or no exposure to IM topics in medical school or residency. Nonetheless, patients are increasingly interested in these approaches, and an increasing body of research findings is allowing their use to become increasingly evidence based.[36] Primary care providers responsibly guide those who seek information and advise them regarding nonallopathic healing approaches.

How can a provider learn more about IM? There are numerous opportunities, but it must be borne in mind that IM is, first and foremost, an overall approach or attitude to providing care. This attitude is rooted in one's personal exploration of health and well-being, and is grounded in awareness of various forms of healing. One example of a curriculum that is designed to facilitate awareness and personal exploration is the Aware Medicine Curriculum of the University of Wisconsin Department of Family Medicine, which longitudinally incorporates self-care, self-reflection, and mindfulness exposure into residency training (point 4 in **Box 4**).

It is also important to acknowledge that the healing arts are just as important as the medical sciences and are in fact 2 parts of the same whole, a point too often forgotten in conventional health care practice. The goal of IM is not merely to add more tools to one's practice toolbox but to refocus on holism, on relationship-centered care, and on optimizing the healing environment as informed by both evidence-based medicine and personal experience grounded in humanism and professionalism.

Medical school, residency, and fellowship training opportunities in IM are rapidly becoming more available. At least 28 medical schools have IM or CAM interest groups, and 22 schools have required coursework. Competencies in IM have also

---

Box 4
How to learn more about IM

1. Connect with local CAM providers. It is not necessary to learn other modalities, although some providers may choose to do so. The key, as in allopathic practice, is to be able to make appropriate referrals. Who are the local health foods and supplement stores? Acupuncturists? Massage therapists? Mindfulness instructors? Chiropractors and osteopaths? Naturopathic doctors? Energy workers? These providers are often thrilled to teach others about what they do and how to collaborate. Discuss credentials, training, experience, and what disorders providers most frequently treat.

2. Build a reference library or list of Web bookmarks. The IM textbook (Rakel D, editor. Integrative medicine, 2nd edition. Philadelphia: Saunders; 2007, available online on MD Consult) is evidence based and offers numerous tools for primary care practice. Chapter 13 of this book lists numerous Web resources one can bookmark and access at the point of care.

3. Consider additional formal training. The Consortium of Academic Health Centers for Integrative Medicine, a group of 44 academic institutions, which offer IM training in various forms, has numerous educational resources and links listed on its Web site (www.imconsortium.org). The Arizona Center for Integrative Medicine offers providers a 2-year fellowship encompassing both residential weeks and online training (http://integrativemedicine.arizona.edu/). The Consortium of Academic Health Centers for Integrative Medicine offers a downloadable 202-page version of its Curriculum in Integrative Medicine: A Guide for Medical Educators at http://www.imconsortium.org/img/assets/20825/CURRICULUM_final.pdf.

4. Become aware of and model other academic programs that incorporate IM themes in medical education. Examples can be found at www.fammed.wisc.edu/integrative and www.fammed.wisc.edu/aware-medicine.

been developed.[37,38] To illustrate recent progress in this area, an Integrative Family Medicine grant, organized by the University of Arizona-Tucson, allowed 6 family medicine residency programs to create 4-year residencies or fellowships with an emphasis on IM. Moreover, opportunities for presently practicing physicians exist, including the Associate Fellowship in Integrative Medicine at the University of Arizona-Tucson and weeklong review courses on IM followed by board examination held by the American Holistic Medical Association.[39] In addition, the Society of Teachers of Family Medicine has an active Integrative Medicine Interest Group for faculty physicians. Instituting IM educational programming in conventional medical settings has led to increased familiarity with and acceptance of IM among providers and other clinic staff.[18]

Educating students, residents, colleagues, and patients is another key element in the role of integrative primary care provider. The authors' clinic group includes postgraduate fellows who participate in the Academic Integrative Medicine Fellowship Program. The group participates in weekly didactic sessions, which are built on a seminar and an experience-based format. Clinic providers and staff are welcome to attend various course offerings also. IM providers also hold interdisciplinary grand rounds on a monthly basis, which include formal IM education and case presentations. Both conventionally trained and CAM practitioners share their professional comments in an open dialog with the group in a way that fosters camaraderie and shared learning. The clinicians also attend on resident teaching services, precept residents at teaching clinics, and participate in medical student clerkships.

SUMMARY

It is essential that health care shift its focus in the direction of prevention, patient-centered care, health-oriented medical teams, and education that includes IM because (1) the demand for primary care continues to increase, (2) patient populations are becoming increasingly active in various alternative and nonconventional forms of medicine, and (3) economic pressures continue to escalate unsustainably from overuse of medical technologies and primary dependence on tertiary care. Whether one is a proponent of IM or not, it is clear that the future of medical care, research, and medical education is moving in this direction. The authors propose several models and suggestions that can be implemented on the clinic level as well as examples of philosophic change that can help inform primary care redesign and positively change the way medicine is practiced in such a way that it improves patient satisfaction, lowers health care cost with emphasis on prevention through wellness, and is based on more patient-practitioner relationship guided treatment options.

REFERENCES

1. Ferrer RL, Hambidge SJ, Maly RC. The essential role of generalists in health care systems. Ann Intern Med 2005;142:691–9.
2. Delva D, Jamieson M, Lemieux M. Team effectiveness in academic primary health care teams. J Interprof Care 2008;22:598–611.
3. Branch WT Jr, Kern D, Haidet P, et al. The patient-physician relationship. Teaching the human dimensions of care in clinical settings. JAMA 2001;286:1067–74.
4. Griffith CH 3rd, Wilson JF, Langer S, et al. House staff nonverbal communication skills and standardized patient satisfaction. J Gen Intern Med 2003;18:170–4.
5. Chez RA, Jonas WB. Toward optimal healing environments in health care. J Altern Complement Med 2004;1:S1–6.
6. Rogers CR. On becoming a person. Boston: Houghton Mifflin; 1995.

7. Hettema J, Steele J, Miller WR. Motivational interviewing. Annu Rev Clin Psychol 2005;1:91–111.
8. Sue DW. Whiteness and ethnocentric monoculturalism: making the "invisible" visible. Am Psychol 2004;59:761–9.
9. Dobie S. Viewpoint: reflections on a well-traveled path: self-awareness, mindful practice, and relationship-centered care as foundations for medical education. Acad Med 2007;82:422–7.
10. Lin CT, Albertson GA, Schilling LM, et al. Is patients' perception of time spent with the physician a determinant of ambulatory patient satisfaction? Arch Intern Med 2001;161(11):1437–42.
11. Lobelo F, Duperly J, Frank E. Physical activity habits of doctors and medical students influence their counseling practices. Br J Sports Med 2009;43:89–92.
12. Brown R. Motivational interviewing, ch 101. In: Rakel D, editor. Integrative medicine. 2nd edition. Philadelphia: Saunders Elsevier; 2007. p. 1065–71.
13. Lancaster T, Stead L. Physician advice for smoking cessation. Cochrane Database Syst Rev 2004;(4):CD000165.
14. Ockene JK. Physician-delivered interventions for smoking cessation—strategies for increasing effectiveness. Prev Med 1987;15(5):723–37.
15. Rakel DP, Hoeft TJ, Barrett BP, et al. Practitioner empathy and the duration of the common cold. Fam Med 2009;41(7):494–501.
16. McKay KM, Imel ZE, Wampold BE. Psychiatrist effects in the psychopharmacological treatment of depression. J Affect Disord 2006;92:287–90.
17. Knight AL, Adelman AM. The family physician and home care. Am Fam Physician 1991;44(5):1733–7.
18. Kligler B, Lebensohn P, Koithan M, et al. Measuring the 'whole system' outcomes of an educational innovation: experience from the integrative family medicine program. Fam Med 2009;41(5):342–9.
19. Rakel DP, Weil A. Philosophy of integrative medicine. In: Rakel DP, editor. Integrative medicine. 2nd edition. Philadelphia: Saunders; 2007. p. 3–13.
20. Barnes PM, Powell-Griner E, McFann K, et al. Complementary and alternative medicine use among adults: United States, 2002. Adv Data 2004;343:1–19.
21. Fineberg H. Welcoming and opening remarks: summit on integrative medicine and the health of the public. Available at: www.imsummitwebcast.org. Accessed January 18, 2010.
22. Schroeder SA. We can do better—improving the health of the American people. N Engl J Med 2007;357:1221–8.
23. American College of Physicians. Joint principles of the patient-centered medical home. Available at: http://www.acponline.org/advocacy/where_we_stand/medical_home/approve_jp.pdf. Accessed September 4, 2008.
24. Antonovsky A. Health, stress and coping. San Francisco (CA): Jossey-Bass; 1979.
25. Jonas WB, Crawford CC. Science and spiritual healing: a critical review of spiritual healing, "energy" medicine, and intentionality. Altern Ther Health Med 2003;9:56–61.
26. Gardner R Jr. The brain and communication are basic for clinical human sciences. Br J Med Psychol 1998;71(Pt 4):493–508.
27. Barrett B, Muller D, Rakel D, et al. Placebo, meaning, and health. Perspect Biol Med 2006;49:178–98.
28. Bandura A. Health promotion by social cognitive means. Health Educ Behav 2004;31:143–64.
29. Meyer B, Pilkonis PA, Krupnick JL, et al. Treatment expectancies, patient alliance, and outcome: further analyses from the National Institute of Mental Health

Treatment of Depression Collaborative Research Program. J Consult Clin Psychol 2002;70:1051–5.

30. Lakhan SE, Laird C. Addressing the primary care physician shortage in an evolving medical workforce. Int Arch Med 2009;2:14.

31. Hall JA, Stein TS, Roter DL, et al. Inaccuracies in physicians' perceptions of their patients. Med Care 1999;37:1164–8.

32. Roter DL, Stewart M, Putnam SM, et al. Communication patterns of primary care physicians. JAMA 1997;277:350–6.

33. Frank E, Breyan J, Elon L. Physician disclosure of healthy personal behaviors improves credibility and ability to motivate. Arch Fam Med 2000;9:287–90.

34. Hart H, Bax M, Jenkins S. Community influences on breast feeding. Child Care Health Dev 1980;6(3):175–87.

35. Li R, Fridinger F, Grummer-Strawn L. Public perceptions on breastfeeding constraints. J Hum Lact 2002;18(3):227–35.

36. National Institutes of Health Health Information Survey 2007. Available at: http://nccam.nih.gov/news/2008/nhsr12.pdf. Accessed January 18, 2010.

37. Kligler B, Maizes V, Schachter S, et al. Education working group, consortium of academic health centers for integrative medicine. Core competencies in integrative medicine for medial school curricula: a proposal. Acad Med 2004;79(6): 521–31.

38. Kligler B, Koithan M, Maizes V, et al. Competency-based evaluation tools for integrative medicine training in family medicine residency—a pilot study. BMC Med Educ 2007;7:7.

39. Maizes V, Silverman H, Lebensohn P, et al. The Integrative family medicine program—an innovation in residency education. Acad Med 2006;81(6):583–9.

Advising Patients About Herbs and Nutraceuticals: Tips for Primary Care Providers

Erica Lovett, MD*, Neelima Ganta, MD

KEYWORDS

- Herbal • Nutraceutical • Dietary supplements
- Integrative medicine
- Complementary and alternative medicine

Herbal remedies and nutraceuticals are used in many households in the United States. According to a 2007 study from the National Center for Complementary and Alternative Health (NCCAM) of the National Institutes of Health (NIH), one third of adults and one tenth of children used some form of complementary and alternative medicine (CAM) within the last month, with herbal and other supplements being the most frequently used CAM modality.[1] Physicians and patients may be interested in natural forms of healing, but they often have differing perspectives. Many health care providers are not comfortable discussing these products, their side effects, or potential interactions with their patients; however, patients desire their physicians to do so. Moreover, patients report using herbals and nutraceuticals regardless of their physician's knowledge base or acceptance of these products.[2] This article discusses basic issues surrounding the use of a number of popular herbs and nutraceuticals other than vitamins and minerals, with the intent of enabling providers to openly discuss their use with patients.

SUPPLEMENT REGULATION IN THE UNITED STATES

Some health care providers are uncomfortable discussing herbal remedies and nutraceuticals with their patients because they did not learn about them in medical school, there are few evidence-based guidelines to guide use, and they are unfamiliar with potential supplement-drug interactions. In addition, the Food and Drug Administration

---

Central Maine Medical Center Family Medicine Residency, 76 High Street, Lewiston, ME 04210, USA
* Corresponding author.
E-mail address: lovetter@cmhc.org (E. Lovett).

Prim Care Clin Office Pract 37 (2010) 13–30
doi:10.1016/j.pop.2009.09.007
0095-4543/10/$ – see front matter © 2010 Elsevier Inc. All rights reserved.

(FDA) does not regulate dietary supplements the way it does medications; providers may not be familiar with supplement manufacturing standards or how to advise patients about choosing different supplement brands.

Some regulation does exist. In 1994, the United States Congress enacted the Dietary Supplements Health and Education Act.[3] This legislation outlines the regulation of herbals, vitamins, minerals, and other "natural health" products. Under the Act, manufacturers have a responsibility to substantiate the safety of their products and make claims about their products only if they are backed by adequate evidence to show that they are not false or misleading. A difference between pharmaceutical regulation and herbal product regulation is that this protection under the Act is postmarketing; manufacturers need not prove safety before distribution. Pharmaceuticals, in contrast, must be FDA approved before sale.

The United States Pharmacopeia (www.usp.org) is an independent, not-for-profit organization that evaluates the effectiveness and safety of herbal products. Although other organizations may provide similar services, no other United States organization that evaluates supplements is recognized under federal law as the nation's official standard-setting body. United States Pharmacopeia standards are enforceable by the FDA.

In 2002, the United States Pharmacopeia designated a voluntary-optional program for manufacturers to obtain the United States Pharmacopeia quality seal. This voluntary program will become mandatory for all companies after 2010. Following current good manufacturing practices is no longer optional as it was in the past for supplement manufacturers. The current good manufacturing practices industry-wide rules require that dietary supplements are manufactured consistently with regards to identity, purity, strength, and composition (no heavy metals); laboratory inspection (sanitation and safety); accurate labeling; and effective release into the body.[4] The new current good manufacturing practices standards are a step in the right direction in providing better-quality, consistent products across all suppliers.

WHO USES SUPPLEMENTS?

The new regulatory standards are essential, given that a significant proportion of the United States population uses dietary supplements. The National Health Survey of 2007 included 23,393 adults 18 years of age and older and 9417 children 17 years of age and younger. According to this survey, 30% to 44% of adults age 18 to 84, 22% of adults 85 and older, and 7% to 16% of children used a CAM therapy within the last month.[1] Nutraceuticals and herbal preparations are the most commonly used therapy in the United States. Nearly 18% of adults and 4% of children in the United States use "nonvitamin, nonmineral, natural products."[1] Other, earlier studies evaluating CAM and supplement use demonstrated similar or slightly higher proportions of individuals (14%–35%) using supplements and herbal therapies.[5,6] The typical adult using CAM is female with a relatively higher income education level.[1] A child's use of CAM is more likely if their parents take supplements, if they are age 12 to 17, if they have more chronic illnesses, or if conventional care is unaffordable.[1]

It is vital for health care providers to ask all patients about dietary supplement use. For instance, it is not uncommon for this author to go on a home visit to a patient who does not fit the previously mentioned characteristics and find a cabinet full of supplements that was never mentioned. Many studies over the last decade substantiate findings that patients are often not comfortable disclosing their supplement use to their physician.[7,8] A 2008 study demonstrated that only half of adult patients and half of patients with chronic health problems disclosed their supplement use.[9]

COMMONLY USED HERBS AND NUTRACEUTICALS

Thousands of different herbs and nutraceuticals are available to consumers. Understandably, care providers cannot be familiar with all of them. One can, however, become familiar with the most popular ones and learn how to advise patients regarding their safety, dosing, and evidence for specific conditions. According to the most recent study from NCCAM, the most commonly-used supplements in adult and pediatric populations include *Echinacea*, fish oil and omega-3 fatty acids, and flaxseed oil. Combinations of supplements are also commonly consumed.[1] Adults also use ginseng, glucosamine, ginkgo, chondroitin, garlic, and coenzyme Q10 (CoQ10), whereas children also take prebiotics and probiotics.[1] The list of the most popular supplements changes over time.

It is also important to know why patients use these supplements. Reasons adults and children use supplements, according to the 2007 NCCAM study, are listed in **Table 1**.

SAFETY ISSUES

Patient safety is also important when deciding how to advise patients regarding specific therapies. This is as true for pharmaceuticals as it is for botanicals and other dietary supplements. Lazarou and coworkers[10] estimated that over 100,000 hospitalized patients died from adverse drug reactions in 1994 alone. It is not clear how many people have been harmed by taking dietary supplements, but the number is thought to be much lower. Case reports regarding supplement adverse effects often fail to

Table 1 Main reasons for dietary supplement use	
Reason	**Percentage**
2007 NCCAM Survey, adults	
Back pain	17.1
Neck pain	5.9
Joint pain	5.2
Arthritis	3.5
Anxiety	2.8
Cholesterol	2.1
Head or chest cold	2
Other musculoskeletal cause	1.8
Severe headache or migraine	1.6
Insomnia	1.4
2007 NCCAM Survey, children	
Back/neck pain	6.7
Head or chest cold	6.6
Anxiety/stress	4.8
Other musculoskeletal cause	4.2
Attention deficit–hyperactivity disorder	2.5
Insomnia	1.8

Data from Barnes PM, Bloom B, Nahin R. Complementary and alternative medicine use among adults and children: United States, 2007. National health statistics reports #12. Hayattsville (MD): National Center for Health Statistics; December 2008.

establish reliable cause-and-effect relationships. To report an adverse event related to a dietary supplement, follow the instructions outlined at the Web site http://www.fda.gov/food/dietarysupplements/alerts/ucm111110.htm. Detailed discussions about supplement safety are found elsewhere.[10,11] The tables that appear in the following sections briefly summarize specific safety and side effect considerations for some of the most popular remedies.

HERBAL THERAPIES

Herbal remedies come directly from different parts of plants, including the roots, stems, flowers, and leaves. Most herbal preparations differ from pharmaceuticals in that they have more than one chemical ingredient, not to mention one or more active compounds, some of which may act synergistically. Some components may help to alleviate side effects of others; many herbalists believe the whole product is much more than its individual parts. Additionally, many other factors affect the potency and efficacy of an herb, such as what time of year it was cultivated, where it was grown, which species was harvested, and what part of the plant is used for standardization.

How an herbal remedy is formulated also influences its effects. Teas, which contain water-soluble compounds, are quite different from extracts obtained using alcohol as a solvent, or dried crude herbs. **Table 2** lists different types of herbal preparations.

READING A SUPPLEMENT LABEL

Understanding the type of preparation and how to read product labels are important factors for advising patients about herbal products. Supplement labels are similar to those for food products. Supplement labels are legally required to include the following: a statement that the product is a supplement, the manufacturer's name and address, a complete list of ingredients, and the net contents of the product.

Good-quality products should also delineate the name of each ingredient; the amount of each ingredient in the product; the serving size and servings per container (note that for some products, a serving is multiple tablets or capsules, which can mislead consumers regarding how long the product lasts); and the percent daily value (normally nothing is established).[12]

Herbal remedies should also list the following: common name and plant name of botanic, plant part used, extract ratio, quantity of starting material and extract, standardization or marker compound, and other ingredients.

The following should be borne in mind when one reads supplement labels. A serving size is designated by the company and is not necessarily a clinically relevant dose. Doses need not be approved by the FDA before marketing. Plant part and extract ratio is important because it too affects the efficacy of the product. The standardization compound is what the industry uses as the basis for claims that each supplement batch contains the same clinically relevant product. For example, alkylamides are used to standardize *Echinacea* and hypericin is used for St John's wort. The label should also contain a lot number in case any safety issues arise with a specific batch of botanicals and an expiration date at which the product is no longer as effective. The expiration date is an estimate, because manufacturers do not all perform stability trials.[12]

Table 3 lists common herbs with dose examples for children and adults. Evidence ratings are included in the third column of **Table 3** for each herb.[13,14]

Table 2 Types of herbal formulations[a]			
Form	**Processing Method**	**Comments**	**Examples**
Crude herb	The whole product is used (flower, stem, root, and so forth)	Provides all of the chemical compounds from a given plant part	Ginger root (nausea)
Water soluble extracts: simple, easy to prepare and cheap	Infusion: steep herb in hot water	Most toxic alkaloids are water insoluble, making teas relatively safe[b]	Chamomile tea (relaxation, colic)
	Decoction: simmer hard parts of plant (roots) for long period of time	Maximum extraction water-soluble parts of plant	Ginseng root (overall tonic)
	Macerate: soak in warm or cold water	Minimizes loss of volatile oils	
Tincture: a solvent extract; made using an organic solvent (usually alcohol or glycerol)	Alcohol is excellent extract for volatile oils, alkaloids, resins, gums, and glycosides	Longer shelf-life Not recommended for alcoholics A 1:5 extract means that 1 g of dried herb is contained in 5 mL of tincture	*Echinacea* (common cold treatment) Osha (male energy enhancement)
Fluid extract (liquid extract)	A more concentrated version of a tincture	Usually a 1:1 or 1:2 ratio (ie, 1 g of dried herb is contained in 1 or 2 mL of the extract)	Saw palmetto (prostatic hypertrophy)
Solid forms (tablets/capsules): most popular form in United States	Solid crude herb: whole herb placed in capsule		Garlic (elevated cholesterol)
	Solid extract: the solvent in a tincture or fluid extract is evaporated to concentrate solids	These are more potent A 5:1 extract has 5 g of the original herb concentrated into just 1 g of solid extract	Gingko (circulation) often studied in dry extract form

[a] Different herbal formulations made from the same plant can contain different chemicals and have different therapeutic and adverse effects. Many herbs are sold in a variety of different forms, and dosing recommendations differ for each. Herbal remedies can also be applied topically, smoked, or used in other forms not described here.
[b] A typical tea recipe is 8 oz of water poured over 2–3 tsp of herb, steeped for 10–15 minutes.
   Data from Rindfleisch JA, Barrett B. Herbs and other dietary supplements. In: Rakel R, editor. Textbook of family medicine. 7th edition. Philadelphia: WB Saunders; 2007.

NUTRACEUTICALS

Other supplements that have been gaining popularity are often referred to as "nutraceuticals." Nutraceuticals, or nutritional supplements, are supplements that are not classified as vitamins, herbs, or minerals. They may be synthesized by the body or isolated from foods or other animal or plant sources.[13] Some claim the body requires more nutraceuticals than it can create, and many nutraceuticals made in the human

Table 3
Common herbs: doses, uses, drug interactions, and cautions

Herb	Dose	Evidence Rating and Common Uses	Drug Interactions	Cautions and Contraindications
American ginseng *Panax quinquefolius*	Tab/cap: 100–200 mg (4% ginsenosides) Decoction: 1–2 g in 150 mL of water Tea: 1.5 g in 5 oz water Whole herb: 0.5–2 g	B Cardiovascular conditions, hyperglycemia, immune system enhancement, type 2 diabetes	ACE inhibitors, warfarin, NSAIDS, aspirin, digoxin, protease inhibitors, nifedipine, methylphenidate, morphine, hormonal therapy, glucose-lowering drugs	Allergy and hypersensitivity Avoid in pregnancy and lactation
Chamomile	Varies depending on condition For gastrointestinal conditions in adults: 2–3 g chamomile, steep in 150 mL hot water, consume 3–4 times daily between meals For children: 1–1.5 g of chamomile, steeped in 150 mL hot water, has been taken 3–4 times daily Infants should not exceed 1 tsp/day; toddlers should not exceed 0.5 C of tea/day; a 50-lb child should not exceed 1 C of tea/day	C Common cold; eczema; diarrhea in children; colic mucositis (from cancer treatment); sleep aid/ sedation Ineffective: postoperative sore throat	Anticoagulant medications (including warfarin); aspirin or aspirin-containing products; NSAIDs; or antiplatelet agents (eg, ticlopidine, clopidogrel, dipyridamole)	Anaphylaxis, allergy and hypersensitivity, children, pregnancy and lactation, avoid 2 wk before dental or surgical procedures, use cautiously if driving or operating machinery
Garlic *Allium sativum*	Tab/cap 600–800 mg/day	B Hyperlipidemia C Antiplatelet effects, antifungal, hypertension, peripheral vascular disease, tick repellant Ineffective: diabetes type II, *Helicobacter pylori*	Warfarin, protease inhibitors thyroid drugs, antihypertensives Avoid use before surgery Avoid large doses during pregnancy and lactation	Allergy and hypersensitivity; bleeding (may increase bleeding); thyroid disorders

Herb	Dosage		Indications	Drug Interactions	Cautions
Ginger *Zingiber officinale*	Adults: 1–2 g/day in divided doses Insufficient evidence for use in children	B C	Hyperemesis gravidarum Chemotherapy-induced nausea and vomiting, inflammation, motion sickness, vertigo	Avoid >1 g/day in pregnancy or before surgery Avoid with gallstones; may be a cholagogue	GRAS by the FDA. Avoid in allergy or hypersensitivity to Zingiberaceae family Reduced nausea from anesthetics, cyclophosphamide May augment anticoagulants May antagonize antacids, reflux drugs
Gingko balboa	Varies depending on condition treated Tab/cap 40–80 mg/day for claudication, up to tid for dementia Effects may take 4–6 wk	A B	Claudication, Alzheimer's disease, dementia Cerebral insufficiency	Warfarin, aspirin, NSAIDS, antiplatelet agents	Allergy and hypersensitivity Avoid with children Avoid during pregnancy and lactation Should be stopped 2 wk before surgery
Echinacea *E purpurea, pallida,* or *angustifolia*	Cap 50–1000 mg	B	Upper respiratory tract infections prevention Upper respiratory infections	Amoxicillin, anesthetics, antineoplastic agents, cytochrome P-450 metabolized agents, corticosteroids, Flagyl	Allergy to Asteraceae/Compositae, atopic reaction, diabetes, AIDS and HIV, hemochromatosis
Milk thistle *Silybum marianum*	Cap: 80–200 mg Tincture: 20–50 mg/kg/24 h IV in divided doses	B C	Chronic hepatitis Cirrhosis Acute viral hepatitis *Amanita phalloides* poisoning	Inhibits cytochromes P-450, 2C6 and 3A4 Inhibits clearance of estrogen Protects liver from damage caused by alcohol, dilantin, acetaminophen, and halothane Protects kidneys from cisplatin	Anaphylaxis, allergy and hypersensitivity, children, pregnancy and lactation, hormone-sensitive cancers

(continued on next page)

Table 3
(continued)

Herb	Dose	Evidence Rating and Common Uses	Drug Interactions	Cautions and Contraindications
Peppermint oil *Menthax piperita L.*	Varies depending on condition treated Adults: 225 mg enteric-coated peppermint oil bid for IBS[15] Children: 0.1–0.2 mL extract in enteric-coated cap po tid[16]	B Antispasmodic Cough Dyspepsia IBS Tension headache (topical)	May have hypoglycemic effect Topical preparations may increase analgesic effect May decrease P-450 3A4 and lead to increased levels of drugs metabolized by this enzyme	GRAS* by FDA May worsen: GERD or achlorhydria, gallbladder disease, G6PD deficiency, hiatal hernia, kidney stones Avoid topical use around facial or chest areas in infants or young children because can induce respiratory difficulties
St John's wort *Hypericum perforatum*	Cap: 100–500 mg SL	A Depression B Somatoform disorder	Triptans, alcohol, anesthetics, antianxiety drugs, antibiotics, warfarin, antidepressants, MAOI, SSRI, TCA, anti-DM agents	Allergy and hypersensitivity, children, pregnancy and lactation
Saw palmetto *Serenoa repens*	Tab/cap: 320 mg Tincture: 2–4 mL Berries: 1–2 g Rectal suppository: 640 mg	A Enlarged prostate C Androgenic alopecia Hypotonic neurogenic bladder	Warfarin, antineoplastic, antihypertensives, blood thinners, antiandrogenic agents	Allergy and hypersensitivity, children, pregnancy and lactation, hormone-sensitive conditions, hypertension, surgical and dental procedures, operating heavy machinery
Valerian root *Valeriana officinalis*	200–400 mg po	C Anxiety, depression, insomnia, menopausal symptoms	Benzodiazepines, barbiturates, antidepressants, β-blockers, St John's Wort	Allergy and hypersensitivity, pregnancy and lactation, operating heavy machinery

Abbreviations: ACE, angiotensin-converting enzyme; AIDS, acquired immune deficiency syndrome; cap, capsule; DM, diabetes mellitus; FDA, Food and Drug Administration; GERD, gastroesophageal reflux disease; GRAS, generally recognized as safe; HIV, human immunodeficiency virus; IBS, irritable bowel syndrome; MAOI, monoamine oxidase inhibitor; NSAID, nonsteroidal anti-inflammatory drug; SL, sublingual; SSRI, selective serotonin reuptake inhibitor; tab, tablet; TCA, tricyclic antidepressant.

Data from Natural Standard, The authority on integrative medicine. Available at: http://naturalstandard.com; and Natural Medicines Comprehensive Database. Available at: http://www.naturaldatabase.com. Both accessed July 5, 2009.

body do decrease with age; however, the value of supplementing with these substances is often unclear.

One popular nutraceutical is CoQ10. CoQ10 is an antioxidant, membrane stabilizer, and cofactor in many metabolic pathways of the body. One action of CoQ10 is to produce energy in the form of ATP in the mitochondria of cells. Humans have the highest levels of CoQ10 in the first 20 years of life, and then it decreases with age. Additionally, some conditions, such as heart failure, further deplete CoQ10. Some authorities suggest supplementing the body's ability to make CoQ10 as one ages, or in cases of heart failure or statin-induced myalgia.[17] CoQ10 helped some heart failure patients feel better but did not change mortality.

Dehydroepiandrosterone (DHEA) is a nutraceutical naturally secreted by the human adrenal gland. DHEA is a precursor for female and male sex hormones. DHEA decreases after age 30 and may be low in people with diabetes, anorexia, end-stage kidney disease, AIDS, and the critically ill. Certain drugs also decrease DHEA (insulin, opiates, corticosteroids, and danazol).[14] Theoretically, supplementing with DHEA could improve symptoms for people with decreased levels. Most studies on DHEA, however, have been short-term, and concern exists that supplementing with DHEA longer than 6 months or in higher than studied amounts (50–100 mg daily) could increase the risk of prostate, breast, and other hormone-sensitive cancers. Supplementing with DHEA can also increase androgen levels and may adversely affect fetal and infant development; DHEA should not be used during pregnancy or lactation.[14]

Omega-3 fatty acids are among the most popular and effective nutraceuticals. Omega-3 fatty acids improve cardiac health by decreasing triglycerides and lowering overall mortality following a myocardial infarction.[17,19,20] The best source of omega-3 fatty acids is fish oil. Some vegetarian sources, such as flaxseed, are promoted as good sources of omega-3 fatty acids. The predominant omega-3 fatty acid in flaxseed is α-linolenic acid, whereas the omega-3 fatty acids in fish oil are predominately docosahexaenoic acid and eicosapentaenoic acid. The human body converts α-linolenic acid to docosahexaenoic acid and eicosapentaenoic acid, but only in small amounts. Flaxseed oil is not as beneficial as fish oil. When flaxseed oil is taken without the seed, the beneficial effects of fiber and lignans, such as improvements in cholesterol, are lost.[13]

Glucosamine and chondroitin are popular nutraceuticals for the treatment of pain from osteoarthritis. Many older studies supported the use of glucosamine for the treatment of pain from mild to moderate osteoarthritis but did not show a great effect from chondroitin.[21] A recent study by the NIH called the Glucosamine/Chondroitin Arthritis Intervention Trial suggested that the combination of glucosamine hydrochloride and chondroitin sulfate decreases pain and prevents progression of pain in patients with moderate to severe knee pain but not those with mild pain.[22] Physiologically, it makes sense that both chondroitin and glucosamine could be beneficial. Both glucosamine and chondroitin are involved with the formation, retention, and repair of cartilage within joints. In some studies, glucosamine sulfate has proved to be more effective than glucosamine hydrochloride.[14] Many integrative providers suggest a 3-month trial of glucosamine sulfate at a dose of 500 mg three times daily for 3 months; the supplement can be continued if the patient believes it is helpful and the cost is not prohibitive.

Table 4 lists common nutraceuticals, uses, common side effects, and drug interactions. Evidence ratings are included in the third column of **Table 4** for each supplement.[13,14]

Table 4
Popular nutraceuticals: uses, side effects, and interactions

Name	Dose[a]	Evidence Rating and Common Uses	Side Effects	Drug Interactions
CoQ10 For hypertension[18]	100–225 mg soft gel capsules/day	A CoQ10 enzyme deficiency B Hypertension (decreases blood pressure by 16–18/10 mm Hg) C Mitochondrial encephalomyopathies, cardiomyopathy, congestive heart failure, HIV-AIDS, migraine headache, muscular dystrophy, after myocardial infarction, Parkinson's disease, periodontal disease, male infertility, statin-induced myopathy Ineffective: diabetes, Huntington's disease	Gastrointestinal, allergic rash in fewer than 1% Side effects minimized by dividing doses >100 mg into two to three doses daily	May increase effects of hypotensive agents Antagonizes warfarin and other anticoagulants Some drugs lower CoQ10 in the body, including some antipsychotics, β-blockers, sulfonylureas, metformin, some statins, and some TCAs
Chondroitin Insufficient evidence for use with children	400 mg tid or 1200 mg/day Full effect may take several weeks Not clear what dose should be used in combination with glucosamine or if both are needed	A Decrease progression of osteoarthritis (knee, low back, finger, knees, hip, tibiofibular, femotibial) and temporomandibular joint disease B Treatment detrussor instability/ urinary incontinence Ineffective: delayed muscle soreness	May increase asthma symptoms Photosensitization, dyspepsia, nausea, diarrhea, constipation, elevated liver enzymes, headache, edema, hair loss, decreased platelet function	May increase effect of anticoagulation medications (NSAIDs, aspirin, warfarin, and so forth) Structurally similar to heparin-avoid in pregnancy

	Dosage	Indications	Adverse Effects	Interactions/Monitoring
DHEA	Adrenal insufficiency: 20–50 mg/day; Depression: 30–90 mg/day; Obesity: 25–100 mg/day; Systemic lupus erythematosis: 20–200 mg/day	B: Adrenal insufficiency, depression, obesity, systemic lupus erythematosis; C: AIDS/HIV, cardiovascular disease, chronic fatigue syndrome, Crohn's disease, fibromyalgia, labor induction, menopausal symptoms, psoriasis, rheumatoid arthritis, sexual dysfunction; Ineffective: memory, muscle strength	Hirsuitism, abnormal menses, emotional changes, headache, and insomnia in women; Acne and aggressive behavior; DHEA can cause elevated levels sex hormones and may increase the risk of prostate, breast, ovarian, and other hormone-sensitive cancers	Many food, drug, and supplement interactions exist; Levels decreased by some drugs: insulin, steroids, opiates, danazol; Levels increased by other drugs: calcium channel blockers, alprazolam; May alter effectiveness of drugs: increased coagulation (decreased effect of warfarin, aspirin, and so forth); Alters cytochrome P metabolism; Decreases effects of methadone; Decreases protective effect of tamoxifen in breast cancer; Monitor thyroid, cholesterol, glucose
Glucosamine Glucosamine is a natural part of healthy cartilage It is not yet clear whether glucosamine sulfate is equivalent to or superior to glucosamine hydrochloride	500 mg tid for 60–90 days Not enough evidence to recommend in children under 18 or during pregnancy or breastfeeding	A: Pain from mild to moderate osteoarthritis of the knee (decrease 0%–20% from baseline); B: Osteoarthritis in other joints; decrease progression of osteoarthritis; C: Rheumatoid arthritis, chronic venous insufficiency, diabetes, temporomandibular joint disorders; Ineffective: hypercholesterolemia	Nausea, reflux, epigastric pain, diarrhea, drowsiness, insomnia; May temporarily increase blood pressure; Palpitations	Contraindications: allergy to shellfish/iodine; Drug interactions: may elevate glucose levels but taking for up to 3 years does not significantly alter glucose or lipid; Can increase effect of Coumadin: monitor INR in anticoagulated patients; Diuretics (eg, furosemide) may increase side effects; Certain supplements may improve efficacy (vitamin C, bromelain, chondroitin sulfate, manganese, fish oil)

(continued on next page)

Table 4
(continued)

Name	Dose[a]	Evidence Rating and Common Uses	Side Effects	Drug Interactions
Fish oil/omega-3 fatty acids	1–6 g/d	A Cardiovascular benefits: Reduces triglycerides (25%–50%) (slight elevation HDL, LDL); decreases blood pressure systolic/diastolic 3.4/2 Patients with h/o myocardial infarction: decrease sudden death, overall mortality, risk of fatal myocardial infarction B Rheumatoid arthritis: improve pain symptoms (morning stiffness and joint tenderness) Eating 2 servings fatty fish weekly decreases risk of developing coronary artery disease Improves response to antidepressants in those with depression and bipolar disorder, including children May improve cognitive function and behavior in children aged 8–12 years with ADD May decrease risk of Alzheimer's disease, certain cancers (colon, rectal, breast, ovarian, oropharyngeal, esophageal)	Halitosis, heartburn, dyspepsia, loose stools, nausea, rash Avoid if shellfish allergy Avoid high doses fatty fish (swordfish, king mackerel, tilefish, and farm-raised salmon) (toxins: mercury, PCBs, dioxins) Freezing, using enteric-coated forms, or taking with meals can minimize side effects Large amounts of mercury in fish can cause multiple neurologic problems Young children should limit consumption no more than 2 oz of fish weekly In pregnancy and breastfeeding avoid certain fish and limit fatty fish to 12 oz per week or about 3–4 servings/wk	Doses >3 g daily can inhibit blood coagulation and increase risk of bleeding may inhibit immune response High doses may inhibit platelets: use caution when using with other medications and herbs that increase bleeding risk May lower blood pressure and have additive effect with antihypertensives Some contraceptives may interfere with triglyceride-lowering effect

	Dose	Evidence/Efficacy	Side Effects	Drug Interactions
Flax Flaxseed oil contains only the α-linolenic acid component of flaxseed, and not the fiber or lignan components[a]	40–50 g/day	C Decreases cholesterol (LDL by 5%–9%, total cholesterol by 8%–18%) Improves menopausal symptoms (decreases hot flashes by 35% and night sweats by 44%) Atherosclerosis, ADD, breast cancer, hyperglycemia, lupus nephritis, obesity, prostate cancer	Bloating, flatulence, abdominal pain, constipation, diarrhea, nausea, dyspepsia High dietary intake α-linolenic acid may increase risk prostate cancer (evidence conflicting) Drink adequate amounts of water when supplementing with flaxseed	May decrease platelet aggregation and increase risk of bleeding when used with aspirin and warfarin May decrease absorption of acetaminophen, ketoprofen, metoprolol, furosemide Antibiotics may limit beneficial effect of lignans in flaxseed May lower blood glucose and increase risk of hypoglycemia with diabetes medications
Lycopene A carotenoid present in many human tissues Lycopene is an antioxidant and antiproliferative substance	Depends on what condition being treated Insufficient evidence to use in children	No grade A or B evidence C Epidemiologic data suggest protective effect against numerous cancers, although a recent study does not support this for breast or prostate cancer Lycopene may be protective for macular degenerative disease, coronary artery disease, hypertension, gingivitis, infertility, and pre-eclampsia. Ineffective: evidence does not support lycopenes use for cell-mediated immune stimulation or lung function after exercise	Diarrhea, dyspepsia, bloating, avoid if known allergy to tomatoes or lycopene May decrease total cholesterol and LDL, increase HDL, decrease blood pressure, may decrease platelet aggregation, may worsen symptoms of gastric ulcers	May interfere with platelet aggregation leading to increased bleeding effect with medications that have similar effect (NSAIDS, aspirin, Coumadin, and so forth) Bile acid sequestrants and statins may decrease lycopene May interfere with tests for prostate cancer May interact with isoflavones

(continued on next page)

Table 4
(continued)

Name	Dose[a]	Evidence Rating and Common Uses	Side Effects	Drug Interactions
Melatonin A naturally occurring neurohormone made in the human pineal gland from the amino acid tryptophan Melatonin increases during dark hours and decreases during daylight	Jet lag: 5 mg melatonin started on the day of travel close to target sleep time at new destination Take every 24 h for several days Insomnia in adults and children: doses from 0.1–5 mg have been used nightly for treating insomnia Some studies have shown no difference in efficacy between low and high doses	A Melatonin treats jet lag B Treats insomnia in adults, elderly, and children Enhances sleep in healthy adults	Diarrhea, headache, abdominal discomfort, drowsiness if taken during daytime There can be an allergic reaction to melatonin (skin rash, autoimmune hepatitis), fatigue, dizziness, headache, mood changes, gynocomastia, decreased sperm count and mobility, may cause changes in intraocular pressures	Drug interactions: may decrease prothrombin time and the effectiveness of warfarin May decrease blood pressure May elevate blood sugar and decrease insulin sensitivity Safety: melatonin is likely safe in doses of 5 mg daily or less over 2 y; melatonin is not safe for women trying to become pregnant or those who are pregnant; melatonin may cause abnormal clotting, especially with patients taking warfarin; overdose may cause disorientation

Probiotics Various strains have been studied; more research needed regarding specific strains and doses for various conditions Most common strains include *Lactobacillus*, *Saccharomyces*, and *Bifidobacterium*	To reduce antibiotic-associated diarrhea: adults, 100 g of probiotic drink bid Continue drink 1 wk after the antibiotics finished 1 capsule of 10^9 colony-forming unit is a standard dose To reduce viral gastroenteritis: children, 3–24 mo, *Saccharomyces boulardii* for 6 d Children 2–47 mo, *Escherichia coli* Nissle 1917 (EcN) solution daily depending on child's weight or *L rhamnosus* strain GG, 1 capsule/day	A Decrease adverse effects of antibiotics including antibiotic-associated diarrhea[24] May decrease growth of *Clostridium difficile* and antibiotic resistance Breast-feeding and pregnant women who take probiotics decrease the risk of their infants developing ectopic eczema[23] Decrease side effects *Helicobacter pylori* treatment (bloating, diarrhea, taste disturbance) Decrease load of *H pylori* and may help eradicate it more completely B Evidence exists for numerous conditions including cirrhosis, colorectal cancer, dental caries, viral diarrhea prevention in children and adults, reduction of symptoms from irritable bowel syndrome, treatment or prevention of diarrhea associated with radiation therapy, decrease recurrent chronic sinusitis, prevention and treatment pouchitis in patients with ulcerative colitis	Most probiotics made from milk; caution when milk allergy is present or use vegan product May produce excessive gas that decreases over time May increase mortality in severe cases of acute pancreatitis	Not enough information available

(continued on next page)

Table 4
(continued)

Name	Dose[a]	Evidence Rating and Common Uses	Side Effects	Drug Interactions
SAMe (S-adenosyl-L-methionine) It is formed in the body by methionine and adenosine triphosphate SAMe is a primary methyl donor in many reactions within the human body	600–1200 mg daily in divided doses for 3 mo in patients with osteoarthritis	B Decreases pain from osteoarthritis C Improvement in depression and fibromyalgia	Safety: 400–600 mg has been safely used for 2 y Higher doses (800–1600 mg) are safe over 1.5 mo May induce hypomania or mania in bipolar patients Not studied in children Side effects: nausea, vomiting, diarrhea, heartburn, skin rash, decreased blood sugar, insomnia, psychomotor excitation	Drug interactions Insulin: SAMe may cause hypoglycemia TCAs: SAMe may cause serotonin syndrome
Soy	Soy extract: 500–1000 mg/day	A Dietary source of protein Lipid-lowering effects B Diarrhea in children	Antibiotics, warfarin, antidiarrheal, antiestrogens, antidiabetes agents	Allergy and hypersensitivity, hormone sensitive malignancies

Abbreviations: AIDS, acquired immune deficiency syndrome; ADD, attention deficit disorder; CFU, colony-forming units; CoQ10, coenzyme Q10; DHEA, dehydroepiandrosterone; HDL, high-density lipoprotein; HIV, human immunodeficiency virus; LDL, low-density lipoprotein; NSAID, nonsteroidal anti-inflammatory drug; TCA, tricyclic antidepressant.

[a] Suggested doses are for specific conditions for each nutraceutical. Please see specific source for more detailed discussions regarding dose and other conditions.

Data from Natural Standard, The authority on integrative medicine. Available at: http://naturalstandard.com; and Natural Medicines Comprehensive Database. Available at: http://www.naturaldatabase.com. Both accessed July 5, 2009.

Box 1
Sources for additional information

Books

Brinckmann J, Wollschlaeger B. In: Blumenthal M, editor. The ABC guide to herbs. 1st edition. Austin (TX): American Botanical Council; 2003.

Rakel D, editor. Integrative medicine. 2nd edition. Philadelphia: WB Saunders; 2007.

Rindfleisch JA, Barrett B. Herbs and other dietary supplements. In: Rakel E, editor. Textbook of family medicine. 7th edition. Philadelphia: WB Saunders; 2007.

Web sites

American Botanic Council (free access): http://abc.herbalgram.org/

National Center for Complementary and Alternative Medicine (free access): http://nccam.nih.gov/health/herbsataglance.htm

National Institute of Health: Office of Dietary Supplements (free access): http://ods.od.nih.gov/Health_Information/Information_About_Individual_Dietary_Supplements.aspx

Naturaldatabase (requires subscription): http://www.naturaldatabase.com.

Natural Standard (requires subscription): http://naturalstandard.com

Food and Drug Administration: Dietary Supplement Information: http://www.fda.gov/Food/DietarySupplements/ConsumerInformation/ucm110567.htm

---

RESOURCES FOR MORE INFORMATION

Often, the key with advising patients regarding dietary supplements is to know where to look up specific information. **Box 1** shows a list of several helpful, evidence-based books and Web sites.

SUMMARY

Herbals and nutraceuticals are part of many patients' daily lives. Many of these products show some benefit, but providers must be mindful of safety issues, including supplement-drug interactions, adverse effects, and product quality. Knowing about different herbal formulations, how to read supplement labels, and where to find additional information about dietary supplements enables health care providers to better counsel their patients regarding safe and appropriate use.

ACKNOWLEDGMENTS

The authors would like to thank Adam Rindfleisch, MD for editing and Kathy Brunjes, MLIS, AHIP - Director Gerrish true Health Sciences Library at CMMC for assistance with final editing of sources.

REFERENCES

1. Barnes PM, Bloom B, Nahin R. Complimentary and alternative medicine use among adults and children: United States 2007. National health statistics reports #12. Hayattsville (MD): National Center for Health Statistics; December 2008.
2. Rindfleisch JA, Barrett B. Herbs and other dietary supplements. In: Rakel R, editor. Textbook of family medicine. 7th edition. Philadelphia: WB Saunders/Elsevier; 2007. p. 243–66.

3. Dietary Supplements Health and Education Act of 1994 (DSHEA), Public Law 103-417, 21 USC 3419.
4. United States Pharmacopeia. Available at: http://www.usp.org/aboutUSP/. Accessed May 15, 2009.
5. Kelly JP, Kaufman DW, Kelley K, et al. Recent trends in use of herbal and other natural products. Arch Intern Med 2005;165(3):281–6.
6. Rogers G. Herb consumers' attitudes, preferences profiled in new market study. Her Geneal 2005;65:60–1.
7. Blendon RJ, DesRoches CM, Benson JM, et al. Americans' views on the use and regulation of dietary supplements. Arch Intern Med 2001;161:805–10.
8. Eisenberg DM, Kessler RC, Van Rampay MI, et al. Perceptions about complementary therapies relative to conventional therapies among adults who use both: results from a national survey. Ann Intern Med 2001;135:344–51.
9. Mehta DH, Gardiner PM, Phillips RS, et al. Herbal and dietary supplement disclosure to health care providers by individuals with chronic conditions. J Altern Complement Med 2008;14(10):1263–9.
10. Lazarou J, Pomerance BH, Corey PN. Incidence of adverse drug reactions in hospitalized patients: a meta-analysis of prospective studies. JAMA 1998;279(15):1200–5.
11. Brinker F. Herb contraindications and drug interactions. 3rd edition. Sandy (OR): Eclectic Publications; 2001.
12. Low Dog T, Barrett M. Botanical medicine: a primer for physicians. University of Arizona. Available at: http://dime.arizona.edu/imres/bot_primer/. Accessed May 20, 2009.
13. Natural Standard. The authority on integrative medicine. Available at: http://naturalstandard.com. Accessed July 5, 2009.
14. Natural Medicines Comprehensive Database. Available at: http://www.naturaldatabase.com. Accessed July 5, 2009.
15. Cappello G, Spezzaferro M, Grossi L, et al. Peppermint oil (Mintoil) in the treatment of irritable bowel syndrome: a prospective double blind placebo-controlled randomized trial. Dig Liver Dis 2007;39(6):530–6.
16. Kline RM, Kline JJ, Di Palma J, et al. Enteric-coated, pH-dependent peppermint oil capsules for the treatment of irritable bowel syndrome in children. J Pediatr 2001;138(1):125–8.
17. Burleson K. Coronary artery disease. In: Rakel D, editor. Integrative medicine. 2nd edition. Philadelphia: Saunders Elsevier; 2007. p. 295–308.
18. Rosenfeldt FL, Haas SJ, Harris CL, et al. Coenzyme Q10 in the treatment of hypertension: a meta-analysis of the clinical trials. J Hum Hypertens 2007;21(4):297–306.
19. Bucher HC, Hengstler P, Schindler C, et al. N-3 polyunsaturated fatty acids in coronary heart disease: a meta-analysis of randomized controlled trials. Am J Med 2002;112:298–304.
20. Din JN, Newby DE, Flapan AD. Omega 3 fatty acids and cardiovascular disease: fishing for a natural treatment. BMJ 2004;328:30–5.
21. Clegg D, Reda DJ, Harris CL, et al. Glucosamine, chondroitin sulfate, and the two in combination for painful knee osteoarthritis. N Engl J Med 2006;354:795–808.
22. Sawitzke AD, Shi H, Finco MF, et al. The effect of glucosamine and/or chondroitin sulfate on the progression of knee osteoarthritis: a report from the glucosamine/chondroitin arthritis intervention trial. Arthritis Rheum 2008;58(10):3183–91.
23. Rosenfeldt V, Benfeldt E, Nielson SD, et al. Effect of probiotic Lactobacillus strains in children with atopic dermatitis. J Allergy Clin Immunol 2003;111:389–95.
24. Van Niel CW, Feudtner C, Garrison MM, et al. Lactobacillus therapy for acute infectious diarrhea in children: a meta-analysis. Pediatrics 2002;109:678–84.

Prescribing Yoga

Meg Hayes, MD[a],*, Sam Chase, MFA, E-RYT[b]

KEYWORDS

• Yoga • Meditation • Movement therapies

Key Points	Evidence Rating	References
Yoga decreases stress and anxiety.	A	1–3
Yoga improves functional status and symptoms in low back pain.	A	4–7
Yoga improves subjective and objective outcomes in asthma.	A	8
Yoga improves oxygen saturation in patients with COPD.	B	
Yoga decreased fatigue in multiple sclerosis patients.	B	9
Yoga is beneficial in patients with eating disorders.	B	10
Yogic breathing may decrease blood pressure.	C	11
Yoga improved physical and quality-of-life measures but not cognitive measures in the elderly.	A	12
Yoga shortens labor duration.	A	13
Yoga improves birth outcomes.	B	14
Yoga improves Rheumatoid Arthritis Disease Activity Score but not quality of life in patients with rheumatoid arthritis.	C	15

The authors have no disclosure to make with respect to funding support.
[a] Oregon Health & Science University, 3181 SW Sam Jackson Park Road, Portland, OR 97239, USA
[b] Sam Chase Yoga, 752 Carroll Street, 1st Floor, Brooklyn, NY 11215, USA
* Corresponding author.
E-mail address: hayesm@ohsu.edu (M. Hayes).

Prim Care Clin Office Pract 37 (2010) 31–47
doi:10.1016/j.pop.2009.09.009
0095-4543/10/$ – see front matter © 2010 Published by Elsevier Inc.

HISTORY

The word *yoga* derives from the Sanskrit word *yuj*, meaning "to yoke, or unite," a root that gives rise to the popular translation of yoga as "union." More broadly understood in a modern context, yoga is a set of principles and practices designed to promote health and well-being through the integration of body, breath, and mind.

Based on depictions of figures in "yoga-like" poses discovered in archeological digs, yoga is thought to have beginnings as early as 3000 BCE, in and around the area that is now India. It is unlikely that the "yoga" then practiced would bear a meaningful resemblance to the yoga we know in the West today. Today's yoga can trace its roots through four periods known as the Vedic period, the Pre-Classical period, the Classical Period, and the Post-Classical period. Each period marks a meaningful shift or transition in the focus and evolution of yoga as we know it now.[16]

During the Vedic period, roughly 2000 BCE–600 BCE, yogic practices centered on surpassing the limitations of the mind, the strong dualist notion of reuniting the physical world with the spiritual world, and studying the Vedas—the elaborate spiritual hymns and rituals of the time, which paid primary attention to the nature of reality and the roots of existence.[16]

The Pre-Classical Period, ranging from 600–200BCE, is marked by the Upanishads, roughly 200 texts that exert heavy influence on later Hindu philosophy, and also by the Bhagavad Gita (written somewhere between 500 and 200BCE), which is considered to be among yoga's oldest written texts. The Gita's 700 verses detail the nature of reality, and the various "yogas" ("karma" or action, "bhakti" or devotion, and "jnana" or wisdom) that can be used to acquire transcendent understanding and liberation. In these texts, the foundations of meditation and the concept of a path to enlightenment begin to emerge strongly.[16]

The Classical Period is anchored by Pantanjali's Yoga Sutras (200 BCE), which attempted to define and standardize yoga through "eight limbs" of study and practice. Patanjali's eight limbs, detailed in **Table 1**, and the underlying philosophy developed in the *Yoga Sutras* came to be called *raja yoga*, from which almost all of modern yoga stems.[16]

The Post-Classical Period following Patanjali is marked by a proliferation of texts, philosophies, and styles that extends from roughly the first century until the late 19th century. During this period, an interest in the study and purification of the physical body emerged to become *hatha yoga*. The primary and most comprehensive treatise of *hatha yoga* comes from Yogi Swatmarama's *Hatha Yoga Pradipika*, written around the 15th century. The advent of *hatha yoga* marks the first serious consideration of the physical exercises that would become today's yoga poses, many of which can be traced back to the *Pradipika* and other concurrent texts.[16]

Yoga in the United States may be said to have its beginning in the late 19th and early 20th centuries, when yoga filtered into the West through the likes of figures such as Swami Vivikenanda who gave a series of highly regarded talks at the 1893 Parliament of Religions in Chicago, and particularly Krishnamacharya, who, although he never left India, was the guru and teacher to several of America's most influential yoga teachers, including B.K.S. Iyengar, Pattabhi Jois, and T.K.V. Desikachar. From the 1940s to the 1980s, prominent Indian figures such as Swami Satchidananda, Swami Sivananda, Yogi Bhajan, Bikram Choudry, and Swami Kripalu brought their unique styles to the West as well, each with a unique and established tradition still in practice today. Since 1990, the landscape of yoga in the West has erupted with diverse styles, teachers, and brand names far beyond the scope of this article to categorize and describe. **Table 2** characterizes key styles currently practiced across the United States.

Table 1
Patanjali's eight limbs

	Sanskrit Name of the Limb	English Translation	Notes
1	The Yamas	Ethical controls	Five moral restraints including *ahimsa* (nonviolence), *satya* (truthfulness), *asteya* (nonstealing), *brahmacharya* (celibacy or sexual discipline), and *aparigraha* (greedlessness).
2	The Niyamas	Ethical observances	Five ethical values including *saucha* (cleanliness), *santosha* (contentment), *tapas* (discipline or austerity), *svadhyaya* (self-study or scriptural study), and *ishvara pranidhana* (surrender to a higher power).
3	Asana	Postures	Originally referring to the seated pose of meditation, but now more broadly referring to the array of physical exercises and postures of the modern yoga practice.
4	Pranayama	Control of vital energy	Pranayama refers to the manipulation of vital energy through the regulation of breath and specific breath exercises, referencing a belief that energy (*prana*) circulates in the body through subtle channels (*nadis*), similar to the more commonly understood Chinese system of *chi* and *meridians*.
5	Pratyahara	Sense-withdrawal	The practice of removing external stimuli and reducing their effects, marked by a mental and sometimes physical isolation or "turning-inward."
6	Dharana	Concentration	The ability to place attention deliberately and hold it indefinitely, which is seen as a foundation and precursor to meditation.
7	Dhayana	Meditation	Mental absorption yielding insight and self-knowledge.
8	Samadhi	Enlightenment	A widely interpreted term variously equated with a state of total mental equilibrium, complete integration between the self and the universe, and bliss.

Table 2
Key yoga styles in the United States

Style	Founder	Current Key Teachers and Centers	Characteristics
Iyengar	B.K.S. Iyengar	B.K.S. Iyengar	A versatile system marked by its attention to precise anatomical alignment within poses, and innovative use of props to allow students to perform poses safely and effectively. Poses are sometimes held for minutes at a time, and always adapted to the level and needs of the student. A therapeutic branch of Iyengar yoga, often called restorative yoga, makes extensive use of props to support students in passive and relaxing poses to promote healing and recovery. Regular Iyengar classes may vary greatly in their content and intensity, depending on the instructor and the level of the group.
Ashtanga	Pattabhi Jois	David Williams, David Swenson, Richard Freeman	Vigorous and highly athletic style, marked by a set sequence of poses. Each pose is performed once and held for 5 breaths, followed by a *vinyasa*—a short series of repeated gestures. A specific *pranayama*—called *ujjayi*, designed to focus the mind and regulate the flow of air, is used throughout a standard 90-minute practice. Classes are taught in two principal styles—either led by an instructor in unison, or in the "Mysore style" where students practice and progress at their own pace within the group while the instructor facilitates each student with verbal and hands-on assistance.
Viniyoga	T.K.V. Desikachar	T.K.V. Desikachar, Gary Kraftsow	A highly therapeutic and usually gentle system, in which poses and practices are adapted to the individual based on the needs of the student and the diagnosis of the teacher. Students flow from pose to pose, holding only briefly. *Pranayama* and chanting are often incorporated throughout.

Style	Founder	Organization	Description
Bikram	Bikram Choudry	Bikram Choudry, Rajashree Choudry	A demanding sequence of 26 poses and two breath exercises, always done in the same order and manner, in a humid room heated to 105 degrees. Each pose is repeated twice, and generally held between 30 and 60 seconds in a standard 90-minute class, known for its rigor and consistency.
Sivananda	Swami Sivananda	International Sivananda Yoga Vedanta Centres	A typically gentle sequence of 13 poses interspersed with periods of supine relaxation. Each pose has multiple variations adaptable to diverse student needs and abilities. Classes regularly include meditation, *pranayama*, and chanting, alongside traditional poses.
Integral	Swami Satchidananda	Swami Ramanada, Integral Yoga Institute, and Yogaville Ashram	A gentle approach similar to Sivananda, Integral offers classes at several levels, each with standard poses moderated with periods of relaxation. In addition to *pranayama*, chanting, and meditation, Integral places great emphasis on the study of traditional yoga texts and selfless service (*karma yoga*).
Kundalini	Yogi Bhajan	Gurmukh Kaur Khalsa, The 3HO Foundation	An energizing practice that blends repetitive gestures with strong breath techniques, meditation, and chanting, with less attention to anatomical precision. Repetitions may last several minutes, making for a very challenging program, but poses are seldom held in stillness for great length. Hands-on adjustment of students is generally not a feature of this style.
Kripalu	Swami Kripalu	Dinabhandu Sarley, The Kripalu Center	A versatile and adaptable practice incorporating breath awareness and self-study with poses. Practices are modified to the individual's goals and needs, and are taught in three stages: first to develop awareness and attention to alignment of the physical body, then in longer holding of poses to challenge the body and mind, and finally as a student-directed "meditation in motion." An open form drawing from many sources, Kripalu classes can vary widely in content and style.

The general trend of yoga in the United States has gravitated toward the physical practices of *asana, pranayama,* and meditation, which have also been the focus of increasing research attention.

ASANA

Asana consists of the physical poses and exercises that were traditionally used as a means to condition and prepare the body for deep and extended periods of meditation, which sometimes involved being seated in stillness for hours or even days. Today, *asana* has become an end in its own right, and the most popular form of yoga practice in the United States. Typical poses range from elementary standing, seated, and supine positions accessible to beginners, to complex and challenging articulations of the body that may be injurious without adequate preparation and strength. Indeed, some poses may be structurally impossible depending on the individual.

PRANAYAMA

Pranayama uses breath exercises to regulate the flow of energy (*prana*) through subtle energy channels (*nadis*) within the body. Various texts mention a number of *nadis* ranging from 72,000 to 350,000, but most acknowledge three distinct *nadis* of primary importance for *pranayama* practice: the *ida* flowing through the left nostril, the *pingala* flowing through the right nostril, and the centrally located *shusumna* running along the spinal cord. *Pranayama* practices to shift and balance the flow of energy in these main channels may also involve cleansing exercises using a sterile string in the nasal passages (*sutra neti*) or a salt water wash (*jala neti*) and rhythmic breathing exercises that condition the respiratory apparatus and cultivate breath awareness.[17]

MEDITATION

Modern meditation practices blend elements described in Patanjali's *dhayana,* and in *dharana* (concentration) and *pratyahara* (sense withdrawal). Traditional Buddhist meditation techniques, such as *metta* (loving kindness) and *vipassana* (insight) meditations may also be included in the study and practice of yogic meditation.[16] Traditional meditation practices often incorporate exercises involving the placement of attention on a *drishti* (focal point), which may include the breath, a chanted or thought mantra, a candle flame, the act of walking, or many others.

STATISTICS ON PRACTICE AND TEACHING

A 2008 "Yoga in America" survey indicates that 15.8 million people in the United States now practice some form of yoga, with an additional 9.4 million reporting that they will "definitely try" yoga within the next year. As an industry, yoga generates roughly 5.7 billion dollars of annual business in the United States, from classes, trainings, media, apparel, and equipment. Nearly half (49.4%) of current practitioners stated they began yoga practice as a means of improving overall health, up from only 5.6% of practitioners in the 2003 survey. Additionally, "one significant trend to emerge from the study is the use of yoga as medical therapy. According to the study, 6.1%, or nearly 14 million Americans, say that a doctor or therapist has recommended yoga to them. In addition, nearly half (45%) of all adults agree that yoga would be a beneficial if they were undergoing treatment for a medical condition."[18]

Traditionally, the practice of yoga was passed from guru to disciple in a personal exchange; advent of group yoga classes, as well as formal group teacher trainings, is a distinctly modern direction in the field. In spite of yoga's increasing popularity and developing validation from evidence-based research, there is at present no legal training requirement to be a yoga teacher in the United States. However, the industry has self-regulated through the formation of the Yoga Alliance, a national body that registers both schools and individual teachers at the 200-hour and 500-hour level, with 200 hours being the recommended minimum for professional teaching. Many teachers choose to pursue thousands of hours of additional training and specialization through continuing education and advanced degrees in related fields such as massage and physical therapy. Yoga Alliance currently lists 19,941 teachers and 875 yoga schools registered nationwide.[19]

THE EMERGENCE OF YOGA AS THERAPY

The rapidly growing field of yoga therapy seeks not only to establish yoga as an independently viable healing practice, but also to integrate yoga into the rubric of currently accepted therapies in the West through participation in, and dissemination of, standardized research studies both within and across disciplines. Writing for the International Association of Yoga Therapists, the largest professional association of yoga therapists with 2300 members, former leader of the Association, Georg Feuerstein, denotes the distinction between yoga and yoga therapy:

> "Yoga therapy is of modern coinage and represents a first effort to integrate traditional yogic concepts and techniques with Western medical and psychological knowledge. Whereas traditional Yoga is primarily concerned with personal transcendence on the part of a 'normal' or healthy individual, Yoga therapy aims at the holistic treatment of various kinds of psychological or somatic dysfunctions ranging from back problems to emotional distress. Both approaches, however, share an understanding of the human being as an integrated body-mind system, which can function optimally only when there is a state of dynamic balance."[20]

Yoga as Medicine, a comprehensive survey of yoga therapy designed for professionals and lay readers alike, identifies 40 research-supported health benefits derived from the practices of *asana* (poses), *pranayama* (breath exercises), and meditation.[21] A comprehensive review of the literature of yoga in medicine provides positive results in a broad range of conditions. However, variability across studies, methodological drawbacks, and sample size limit the extent to which yoga can be deemed effective from an evidence-based perspective. However, given the benefits, further research in this area is certainly warranted. Future research should examine what components of yoga are most beneficial, and what types of patients receive the greatest benefit from yoga interventions.

People who practice yoga note that it contributes to happiness, finding meaning in life, and feeling connected to others. The practice can be an excellent aerobic and weight-bearing exercise program, helping practitioners to regulate breathing, decrease stress, and improve quality of life. All of these factors are positive attributes for a person who desires to maintain good health or to improve health. These attributes make it more likely that a person will be able to affect lifestyle changes such as cutting back or eliminating tobacco use, alcohol, or drugs; make healthier food choices and eat appropriate amounts of food rather than overeating; and turn to yoga practice for stress reduction. All of these considerations are important in creating and maintaining a healthy lifestyle. How specifically does yoga help improve health problems? Although the research into yoga as medicine is in its infancy, there is a large body of work in India, and developing scientific inquiry in the West to help us understand more about this practice as medicine. Increased scientific investigation of yoga would help us to understand better how to use this treatment modality in the US health system. Many studies to date have provided promising pilot and preliminary data that deserve further inquiry. Appropriately powered studies, the use of technology such as physiologic studies, immune modulators, functional MRI and positron emission tomography (PET) scans, as well as long-term investigations will help us to understand the therapeutic value of yoga practice and the mechanism of action.

CHARACTERISTICS OF YOGA USERS

To characterize yoga users, medical reasons for use, perceptions of helpfulness, and disclosure of use to medical professionals Birdee and colleagues[23] looked at cross-sectional survey data from the 2002 National Health Interview Survey (NHIS) Alternative Medicine Supplement (n = 31044) to examine correlates of yoga use for health. The estimated prevalence from 2002 NHIS of yoga for health was 5.1% corresponding to more than 10 million adults. Yoga users were predominately white and female, and college educated with a mean age of 39.5 years. The medical conditions most commonly associated with yoga use were musculoskeletal conditions, mental health conditions, sprains, and asthma. Chronic obstructive pulmonary disease (COPD) and hypertension were also associated with yoga use, but to a lesser degree. Most users reported yoga to be helpful for their medical conditions, especially for musculoskeletal and mental health concerns, and 61% reported that yoga was important in maintaining health, yet only 25% disclosed yoga use to their physician.

STRESS MANAGEMENT

Generalized anxiety disorder (GAD) is common, with 12-month and lifetime prevalence rates, based on DSM-IV criteria, estimated at 2.1% and 4.1%, respectively.[24] The prevalence is estimated to be between 5% and 8% in the primary care setting.[25,26] Twice as many women as men have the disorder.[27] The number of office visits with a recorded anxiety disorder diagnosis increased from 9.5 million in 1985, to 11.2 million per year in 1993 to 1994 and 12.3 million per year in 1997 to 1998, accounting for 1.9%, 1.6%, and 1.5% of all office visits in those years, respectively.[27]

Any number of daily stressors can activate the neurotransmitters norepinephrine, serotonin, gamma-aminobutyric acid (GABA), and cortisol, causing the pupils to dilate, the heart to beat faster and harder, sweating, increased blood pressure, and shunting of blood away from the abdominal organs to the large muscle groups. During the stress response, white cells marginate, platelets aggregate, and stored energy sources are mobilized through activation of the sympathetic nervous system. Once the stressful stimulus has passed, the parasympathetic nervous system restores this mobilization to a more restful state. However, in our modern society of near constant stress of overwork, unemployment, economic concerns, family challenges, traffic, disturbing news of world events, and so forth, the stress response may be turned on repeatedly and for extended periods of time for conditions that rarely demand the physical response that the mobilization of the sympathetic nervous system was designed to support. Yoga practice can help to modulate the stress response in a number of ways. The inward focus of yoga can help to quiet the external stimuli that may be driving the stress response. The relaxed breathing used in yoga practice modulates the physiologic triggers that initiate the sympathetic cascade.

Several studies on special patient populations undergoing stress and anxiety provide evidence for the efficacy of yoga practice for modulating the stress response. One study looking at the effect of integrated yoga practice and guided yogic relaxation on perceived stress and measured autonomic response in healthy pregnant women found that perceived stress decreased by 31.57% in the yoga group and increased by 6.60% in the control group ($P = .001$). During a guided relaxation period in the yoga group, compared with values obtained before a practice session, the high-frequency band of the heart rate variability spectrum (parasympathetic) increased by 64% in the 20th week and by 150% in the 36th week, and both the low-frequency band (sympathetic) and the low-frequency to high-frequency ratio were concomitantly reduced ($P < .001$ between the two groups). Moreover, the low-frequency band remained decreased after deep relaxation in the 36th week in the yoga group.[1]

Another study looking at the effects of an integrated yoga program on cortisol rhythm and mood states in early breast cancer patients undergoing adjuvant radiotherapy revealed significant decreases in anxiety, depression, perceived stress, and salivary cortisol compared with controls.[2]

A three-armed controlled study to look at the ability of yoga and meditation to alleviate stress, anxiety, mood disturbance, and musculoskeletal problems in professional musicians found a trend toward less music performance anxiety and significantly less general anxiety, tension, depression, and anger at the end of the intervention relative to controls.[3]

LOW BACK PAIN

Specific schools of yoga may be particularly beneficial for chronic low back pain. A randomized trial of 101 patients with chronic low back pain found viniyoga (12 weekly 75-minute sessions) improved functional status and symptoms at 12 weeks compared with two other interventions: a back exercise class, or a self-care book; at 26 weeks outcomes for yoga were equivalent to exercise but remained superior to the self-care book. Yoga was associated with decreased medication use compared with exercise or the self-care book. The yoga program combined breathing techniques, simple yoga postures, and deep relaxation.[4] Smaller trials comparing Iyengar yoga to exercise instruction or standard exercise were inconclusive, although suggested a trend of improvement for the yoga participants.[5,6]

A wait-list randomized controlled trial (RCT)demonstrated that short-term, intensive yoga therapy reduced pain-related disability and improved spinal flexibility in patients with chronic low back pain better than a physical exercise regimen.[7] The study matched the yoga intervention and physical exercise groups for time on intervention and attention. The intervention consisted of a 1-week intensive residential program of asanas designed for back pain and included pranayamas, meditation, and didactic and interactive sessions on the philosophy of yoga. Pain-related outcomes were assessed by the Oswestry Disability Index (ODI) and by spinal flexibility, which was assessed using a goniometer at pre- and postintervention. There was a significant reduction in ODI scores in the yoga group compared with the control group. Spinal flexibility measures improved significantly in both groups but the yoga group had greater improvement as compared with controls on spinal flexion, spinal extension, and right and left lateral flexion.

ASTHMA AND CHRONIC OBSTRUCTIVE PULMONARY DISEASE

Because yoga practice improves posture, lengthens the spine, develops strength and flexibility of muscles, and involves breathing exercise, there has been a great deal of attention to the value of yoga in improving outcomes for patients with obstructive breathing problems. There is a developing body of evidence on the efficacy of yoga in the management of bronchial asthma. Many studies have reported significant improvements in pulmonary function testing, quality of life, and reduction in airway hyperreactivity, decreased frequency of attacks, and medication use for asthma patients in yoga intervention studies.

A recent randomized controlled study comparing conventional care to conventional care plus yoga attempted to understand the immunological mechanisms by which yoga improves outcomes in bronchial asthma. The study demonstrated steady and progressive improvement in pulmonary function, the change being statistically significant in the case of the first second of forced expiratory volume (FEV1) at 8 weeks, and peak expiratory flow rate (PEFR) at 2, 4, and 8 weeks as compared with the corresponding baseline values. There was a significant reduction in exercise-induced bronchoconstriction in the yoga group. However, there was no corresponding reduction in the urinary prostaglandin D2 metabolite levels in response to the exercise challenge, and no significant change in serum eosinophilic cationic protein levels during the study period in either group. There was a significant improvement in Asthma Quality of Life (AQOL) scores and decrease in rescue medication use in both groups with improvement achieved earlier and more completely in the yoga group than the control group for both parameters. The researchers conclude that adding the mind body approach of yoga conventional care results in measurable improvement in subjective and objective outcomes in bronchial asthma, although the mechanism of action with respect to immune modulation has not been elucidated.[8]

In a pilot study to evaluate the safety, feasibility, and efficacy of yoga training as an effective exercise strategy to manage the symptom of dyspnea in patients with COPD, the end points of decreasing dyspnea intensity (DI) and dyspnea-related distress (DD) in older adults with COPD was undertaken. The subjects, elderly patients with COPD, participated safely in a 12-week yoga program especially designed for patients with COPD. After the program, the subjects tolerated more activity with less DD and improved their functional performance 6-minute walk test and small positive changes in muscle strength and health-related quality of life.[28]

Another study investigated the ability to improve gas exchange in COPD patients with yoga breathing, as it had previously been reported in patients with chronic heart failure and in participants exposed to high-altitude hypoxia. COPD patients without previous yoga practice and taking only short-acting beta2-adrenergic blocking drugs were enrolled. Plethysmography during 30-minute spontaneous breathing at rest and during a 30-minute yoga lesson was conducted to study ventilatory pattern and oxygen saturation. During the yoga lesson, the patients were requested to mobilize in sequence the diaphragm, lower chest, and upper chest adopting a slower and deeper breathing. The oxygen saturation (SaO2%), was significantly improved with all participants reporting comfort during the yoga practice and no increase in dyspnea.[29]

MULTIPLE SCLEROSIS

In a 6-month trial comparing weekly Iyengar yoga with home practice, weekly exercise on stationary bicycle with home exercise program, and a wait-list control group, patients with clinically definite multiple sclerosis and expanded disability status score of 6 or less were randomly assigned. The subjects in the yoga group and the exercise group demonstrated significant improvement in fatigue as measured by the Multi-Dimensional Fatigue Inventory and Short Form-36 compared with wait-list controls, with no adverse events related to the intervention reported.[9]

EATING DISORDERS AND OBESITY

A 12-week yoga program aimed at reducing binge eating severity randomized a community-based sample of women between 25 and 63 years of age who identified with diagnostic criteria for binge eating disorder (BED) and a body mass index (BMI) greater than 25. The trial was undertaken assigning participants to yoga or wait-list control groups. Primary outcomes included the Binge Eating Scale (BES) and International Physical Activity Questionnaire (IPAQ). Secondary outcomes comprised measures for BMI, hips, and waist. For the yoga group, self-reported reductions in binge eating and increases in physical activity were statistically significant. Small yet statistically significant reductions for BMI, hips, and waist measurement were obtained. The wait-list control group did not improve significantly on any measures.[10]

HYPERTENSION

Breathing exercises practiced in various forms of yoga are thought to influence autonomic function and therefore may improve hypertension. In a randomized, prospective, controlled study, male and female patients aged 20 to 60 years with stage 1 essential hypertension were randomly and equally divided into the control and two intervention groups, who were advised to do 3 months of slow-breathing and fast-breathing exercises, respectively. Slow breathing had a stronger effect than fast breathing with blood pressure decreased longitudinally over a 3-month period with both interventions. Autonomic function testing including standing-to-lying ratio (S/L ratio), immediate heart rate response to standing (30:15 ratio), valsalva ratio, heart rate variation with respiration (E/I ratio), hand grip test and cold presser response showed significant change in only the slow breathing group. This suggests that improvement in both sympathetic and parasympathetic reactivity may be the mechanism associated with blood pressure improvement in the slow breathing group.[11]

STRENGTH AND BALANCE IN THE ELDERLY

A major source of morbidity and mortality in the elderly population is loss of strength and balance. This is particularly notable in performance of activities of daily living and in falls that can result in significant injury including hip fracture and subdural hematoma. In a study to look at cognitive function in healthy men and women aged 65 to 85 years, participants were randomized to 6 months of Hatha yoga class, walking exercise, or wait-list control. Those in the intervention groups were also asked to practice at home. Although there were no effects from either of the active interventions on any of the cognitive and alertness outcome measures, the yoga intervention produced improvements in physical measures such as timed 1-legged standing and forward flexibility as well as a number of quality-of-life measures related to sense of well-being and energy and fatigue compared with controls. Those in the yoga group showed significant improvement in quality-of-life and physical measures compared with exercise and wait-list control groups.[12] In addition to strength, flexibility, and balance, yoga is a weight-bearing activity that can improve bone density, also leading to decreased fracture risk.

PREGNANCY

Prenatal yoga classes have become popular throughout the country as a means of diminishing pregnancy-associated back and pelvic pain, as well as strengthening the core musculature in preparation for childbirth. The meditative quality of yoga might

---

Box 1
Selected resources for practitioners and professionals

ASANA

Iyengar, B.K.S. *Light on Yoga*. New York: Schocken Books, 1966.

Mittra, Dharma. *Asanas: 608 Yoga Poses*. Novato: Here + There, 2003.

PRANAYAMA

Iyengar, B.K.S. *Light on Pranayama: The Yogic Art of Breathing*. Chestnut Ridge: Crossroad Publishing, 1985.

Rama, Swami; Ballentine, Rudolph MD; & Hymes, Allan MD. *Science of Breath: A Practical Guide*. Honesdale: Himalayan Institute, 1979.

Rosen, Richard. *Pranayama Beyond the Fundamentals: An In-Depth Guide to Yogic Breathing*. Boston: Shambala, 2006.

MEDITATION

Ballantine, Rudolph MD. *Theory and Practice of Meditation*. Honesdale: Himalayan Institute, 1987.

Khalsa, Dharma Singh MD; Stauth, Cameron. *Mediation as Medicine*. New York: Atria, 2002.

Salzberg, Sharon. *Insight Meditation: A Step-by-Step Course on How to Meditate*. Louisville: Sounds True, 2006.

YOGA THERAPY

The International Association of Yoga Therapists: http://www.iayt.org

Payne, Larry PhD; Usatine, Richard MD. *Yoga RX: A Step-by-Step Program to Promote Health, Wellness, and Healing for Common Ailments*. New York: Broadway Books, 2002.

McCall, Timothy MD. *Yoga as Medicine: The Yogic Prescription for Health and Healing*. New York: Bantam Dell, 2007.

IYENGAR

Iyengar Yoga: National Association of the United States: http://www.iynaus.org

Iyengar, B.K.S. *The Tree of Yoga*. Boston: Shambala, 1988

Iyengar, B.K.S. *Yoga: The Path to Holistic Health*. London: Dorling Kindersley, 2001

ASHTANGA

Ashtanga Yoga: http://www.ashtanga.com

Jois, Sri K. Pattabhi. *Yoga Mala*. New York: North Point Press, 1999.

Swenston, David. *Ashtanga Yoga: The Practice Manual*. Austin: Ashtanga Yoga Productions, 2007.

VINIYOGA

The American Viniyoga Institute: http://www.viniyoga.com

Desikachar, T.K.V. *The Heart of Yoga: Developing a Personal Practice*. Rochester: InnerTraditions, 1999.

Kraftsow, Gary. *Yoga for Wellness: Healing with the Timeless Teachings of Viniyoga*. NewYork: Penguin, 1999.

BIKRAM

Bikram's Yoga College of India: http://www.bikramyoga.com

Choudhury, Bikram. *Bikram's Beginning Yoga Class*. New York: Tarcher/Putnam, 2000.

SIVANANDA

International Sivananda Yoga Vedanta Centres: http://www.sivananda.org

The Sivananda Yoga Center. *The Sivananda Companion to Yoga: A Complete Guide to the Physical Postures, Breathing Exercises, Diet, Relaxation, and Meditation Techniques of Yoga.* New York: Fireside, 1983.

INTEGRAL

Integral Yoga International: http://www.iyiva.org

Oakville Ashram: http://www.yogaville.org

Satchidananda, Swami. *Integral Yoga Hatha.* Yogaville: Satchidananda Ashram, 1970.

KUNDALINI

The Kundalini Research Institute: http://www.kriteachings.org

The 3HO Foundation: http://www.3ho.org

Khalsa, Dharam Singh; O'Keefe, Darryl. *The Kundalini Yoga Experience: Bringing Body, Mind, and Spirit Together.* New York: Fireside, 2002.

KRIPALU

The Kripalu Center: http://www.kripalu.org

Faulds, Richard. *Kripalu Yoga: A Guide to Practice On and Off the Mat.* New York: Bantam, 2005.

also be used to cope with pregnancy- and birth-associated anxiety, and to increase the ability to focus and manage labor-associated pain.

A recent randomized study conducted in Thailand examined the effects of a yoga program during pregnancy on maternal comfort, labor pain, and birth outcomes. The yoga program involved six, 1-hour sessions at prescribed weeks of gestation. The intervention group was found to have higher levels of maternal comfort during labor and 2-hours postpartum, and experienced less subjective labor pain than the control group. In each group, pain increased and maternal comfort decreased as labor progressed. No differences were found between the groups regarding pethidine medication usage, labor augmentation, or newborn Apgar scores at 1 and 5 minutes. The intervention group was found to have a shorter duration of the first stage of labor, as well as the total time of labor.[13]

The effect of yoga on pregnancy outcomes was studied in a prospective, matched, observational study of women enrolled between 18 and 20 weeks gestational age. Women were matched for age, parity, body weight, and Doppler velocimetry scores of umbilical and uterine arteries. Yoga practices, including physical postures, breathing, and meditation were practiced by the yoga group 1 hour daily, from the date of entry into the study until delivery. The control group walked 30 minutes twice a day (standard of care at the study site) during the study period. Compliance was closely followed for both groups with frequent telephone calls and maintenance of an activity diary. Primary outcomes of birth weight and preterm labor were significantly improved in the intervention group. In addition, complications such as isolated intrauterine growth retardation (IUGR) and pregnancy-induced hypertension (PIH) with associated IUGR were also significantly lower in the yoga group. There were no significant adverse effects noted in the yoga group. This study suggests that inclusion of prenatal yoga during the second and third trimesters may improve birth outcomes.[14]

RHEUMATOID ARTHRITIS

Disease activity over time produces functional disability in patients with rheumatoid arthritis (RA). The Disease Activity Score (DAS-28) is a quantification of functional status in RA that is used in clinical trials. The DAS-28 includes measurement of the number of joints tender to the touch, number of swollen joints, the erythrocyte sedimentation rate (ESR) and patient assessment of disease activity. The Health Assessment Questionnaire (HAQ) is the most common assessment tool for functional disability. A pilot study of 12 sessions of a Raj yoga program on RA disease activity compared with controls demonstrated significant improvements in the RA DAS-28 and HAQ, however there was no demonstrated improvement in quality of life.[15]

MENOPAUSE

A recent systematic review of the efficacy of yoga for treatment of menopausal symptoms concluded that the evidence is insufficient to suggest that yoga is an effective intervention for menopause. Further research is recommended to investigate whether there are specific benefits of yoga for treating menopausal symptoms.[30]

However, a recent pilot study provided promising support for the beneficial effects of a comprehensive yoga program for hot flashes and other menopausal symptoms in early-stage breast cancer survivors. These patients have limited options for the treatment of hot flashes and related symptoms. In addition, therapies widely used to prevent recurrence in survivors, such as tamoxifen, tend to induce or exacerbate menopausal symptoms. In this RCT, early-stage breast cancer (stages IA–IIB) survivors who were experiencing hot flashes were randomized to an 8-week Yoga of Awareness program (gentle yoga poses, meditation, and breathing exercises) or to wait-list control. The primary outcome was daily reports of hot flashes collected at baseline, posttreatment, and 3 months after treatment via an interactive telephone system. Data were analyzed by intention to treat. At posttreatment, women who received the yoga program showed significantly greater improvements relative to the control condition in hot-flash frequency, severity, and total scores and in levels of joint pain, fatigue, sleep disturbance, symptom-related bother, and vigor. At 3-month follow-up, patients maintained their treatment gains in hot flashes, joint pain, fatigue, symptom-related bother, and vigor and showed additional significant gains in negative mood, relaxation, and acceptance.[31]

PRESCRIBING YOGA AND HOW TO FIND A TEACHER

For the physician prescribing yoga, care in finding and referring to appropriate yoga studios and instructors is required. Because no form of teacher accreditation currently exists, and because of the breadth of technique both within and among traditions, the patient pursuing yoga as a therapeutic modality should consider the various kinds of yoga available, as well as the experience of the teacher in designing and adapting a yoga practice that will maximize the positive impact a yoga practice will have for the patient.[22] Particularly for practitioners seeking to address a medical condition or physicians seeking to refer a patient, personal knowledge of both the teacher and the tradition is of paramount importance. The tradition of yoga has always held personal inquiry and experience as its highest currency, and prospective students of yoga would do well to evaluate potential teachers and studios based on their level of training, areas of expertise, standing in the field, and the quality of the teacher-student connection before committing to a practice.

Class sizes can range from a single student to several hundred. Although therapeutic sessions are generally conducted on a one-on-one basis or in very small groups to maximize the interaction between therapist and client, large group classes may include little if any individual attention or tailoring to medical concerns, and open classes not specifically geared toward beginning students or those with health issues may assume that the practitioner has appropriate knowledge of form, modifications, and contraindications. Many teachers and studios offer specialized instruction for specific communities and conditions, including classes for elderly, cancer patients, prenatal women, and blind people.

Cost varies equally widely. Yoga was historically taught for free, and among some teachers and studios continues to be free or donation based. However, it is more common to see group classes ranging anywhere from $10 to $25 per person, with price breaks for purchase of a package of classes or over a period of time, and private instruction ranging anywhere from $50 to hundreds of dollars per hour. There is currently no insurance reimbursement for yoga.

The frequency and span of an ideal practice depends greatly on the condition of the practitioner, and in particular the nature of any medical issues present during the practice. Several traditions, notably Bikram and Ashtanga, encourage daily practice with periodic days of rest, whereas others invite the students to develop their own schedules in accordance with their needs and desires. Because yoga comprises not only a system of healing, but also a maintenance system, yoga practice can become an enduring and lifelong journey designed to grow and adapt with the changing individual. Consistency is key, and the benefits of a well-designed personal practice have been shown to be cumulative over time.[22] Selected resources for practitioners and professionals are shown in **Box 1**.

REFERENCES

1. Satyapriya M, Nagendra H, Nagarathna R, et al. "Effect of integrated yoga on stress and heart rate variability in pregnant women". Int J Gynaecol Obstet 2009;104(3):218–22.
2. Vadiraja H, Raghavendra R, Nagarathna R, et al. "Effects of a yoga program on cortisol rhythm and mood states in early breast cancer patients undergoing adjuvant radiotherapy: a randomized controlled trial". Integr Cancer Ther 2009;8(1): 37–46.
3. Khalsa S, Shorter S, Cope S, et al. "Yoga ameliorates performance anxiety and mood disturbance in young professional musicians". Appl Psychophysiol Biofeedback 2009;34(4):279–89.
4. Sherman KJ, Cherkin DC, Erro J, et al. Comparing yoga, exercise, and a self-care book for chronic low back pain: a randomized, controlled trial. Ann Intern Med 2005;143:849.
5. Galantino ML, Bzdewka TM, Eissler-Russo JL, et al. The impact of modified Hatha yoga on chronic low back pain: a pilot study. Altern Ther Health Med 2004; 10:56.
6. Williams KA, Petronis J, Smith D, et al. Effect of Iyengar yoga therapy for chronic low back pain. Pain 2005;115:107.
7. Tekur P, Singphow C, Nagendra H, et al. "Effect of short-term intensive yoga program on pain, functional disability and spinal flexibility in chronic low back pain: a randomized control study". J Altern Complement Med 2008;14(6):637–44.

8. Vempati R, Bijlani RL, Deepak K, et al. "The efficacy of a comprehensive lifestyle modification programme based on yoga in the management of bronchial asthma: a randomized controlled trial". BMC Pulm Med 2009;9(1):37.

9. Oken B, Kishiyama S, Zajdel D, et al. "Randomized controlled trial of yoga and exercise in multiple sclerosis". Neurology 2004;62(11):2058–64.

10. McIver S, O'Halloran P, McGartland M, et al. "Yoga as a treatment for binge eating disorder: a preliminary study". Complement Ther Med 2009;17(4):196–202.

11. Mourya M, Mahajan A, Singh N, et al. "Effect of slow- and fast-breathing exercises on autonomic functions in patients with essential hypertension". J Altern Complement Med 2009;15(7):711–7.

12. Oken BS, Zajdel D, Kishiyama S, et al. "Randomized, controlled, six-month trial of yoga in healthy seniors: effects on cognition and quality of life". Altern Ther Health Med 2006;12(1):40–7.

13. Chuntharapat S, Petpichetchian W, Hatthakit U, et al. "Yoga during pregnancy: effects on maternal comfort, labor pain and birth outcomes". Complement Ther Clin Pract 2008;14(2):105–15.

14. Narendran S, Nagarathna R, Narendran V, et al. "Efficacy of yoga on pregnancy outcome". J Altern Complement Med 2005;11(2):237–44.

15. Badsha H, Chhabra V, Leibman C, et al. "The benefits of yoga for rheumatoid arthritis: results of a preliminary, structured 8-week program". Rheumatol Int 2009;29(12):1417–21.

16. Feuerstein G. The yoga tradition: its history, literature, philosophy and practice. Prescott (AZ): Hohm Press; 2001. p. 91–138, 155–82, 213–38, 381–426.

17. Rama S. Portal to higher awareness. In: Ballentine R, Hymes A, editors. Science of breath: a practical guide. Honesdale: Himalayan Institute; 1979. p. 72–112.

18. Yoga in America Study. Available at: http://www.yogajournal.com/press/yoga_in_america. Accessed August 21, 2009.

19. Yoga alliance database search. Available at: http://www.yogaalliance.org/school_search.cfm. Accessed August 25, 2009.

20. Contemporary definitions of yoga therapy. Available at: http://www.iayt.org/siet_Vx2/publications/articles/defs.htm. Accessed August 25, 2009.

21. McCall T. The science of yoga. In: Yoga as medicine. New York: Bantam Dell; 2007. p. 26–47.

22. McCall T. Choosing a style of yoga and a teacher. In: Yoga as medicine. New York: Bantam Dell; 2007. p. 102–20, 120–129.

23. Birdee GS, Legedza A, Saper R, et al. "Characteristics of yoga users: results of a national survey". J Gen Intern Med 2008;23(10):1653–8.

24. Grant BF, Hasin DS, Stinson FS, et al. Prevalence, correlates, co-morbidity, and comparative disability of DSM-IV generalized anxiety disorder in the USA: results from the National Epidemiologic Survey on alcohol and related conditions. Psychol Med 2005;35:1747.

25. Roy-Byrne PP, Katon W. Generalized anxiety disorder in primary care: the precursor/modifier pathway to increased health care utilization. J Clin Psychiatry 1997;58(Suppl 3):34.

26. Kroenke K, Spitzer RL, Williams JB, et al. Anxiety disorders in primary care: prevalence, impairment, comorbidity, and detection. Ann Intern Med 2007;146:317.

27. Harman JS, Rollman BL, Hanusa BH, et al. Physician office visits of adults for anxiety disorders in the United States, 1985–1998. J Gen Intern Med 2002;17:165.

28. Donesky-Cuenco D, Nguyen H, Paul S, et al. "Yoga therapy decreases dyspnea-related distress and improves functional performance in people with chronic

obstructive pulmonary disease: a pilot study". J Altern Complement Med 2009; 15(3):225–34.

29. Pomidori L, Campigotto F, Amatya T, et al. "Efficacy and tolerability of yoga breathing in patients with chronic obstructive pulmonary disease: a pilot study". J Cardiopulm Rehabil Prev 2009;29(2):133–7.

30. Lee M, Kim J, Ha J, et al. "Yoga for menopausal symptoms: a systematic review". Menopause 2009;16(3):602–8.

31. Carson J, Carson K, Porter L, et al. "Yoga of awareness program for menopausal symptoms in breast cancer survivors: results from a randomized trial". Support Care Cancer 2009;17(10):1301–9.

An Introduction to Clinical Research in Osteopathic Medicine

Brian E. Earley, DO[a],*, Helen Luce, DO[a,b]

KEYWORDS

- Osteopathic medicine • Research • OMT • OMM
- Manipulation • Risks

Osteopathic medicine encompasses a unique philosophy, distinct diagnostic methods, and complementary manipulative treatment that sets it apart from allopathic medicine. Osteopathic medicine is the smaller of the 2 schools of medicine in the United States, but the number of Doctors of Osteopathic Medicine (DOs) is increasing at a higher rate than allopathic physicians (MDs).[1] This article introduces osteopathic medicine, including a brief history, education requirements, philosophy, and potential risks of OMT (osteopathic manipulative treatment). The main body of this article focuses on difficulties associated with conducting osteopathic research and provides an overview of available studies, which have researched the effect of OMT on various conditions.

HISTORY

Andrew Taylor Still, the founder of osteopathic medicine, was the son of a Methodist minister and pioneer physician. His fascination with human anatomy and the science of healing influenced him to become a physician. As a typical frontier physician, he had to deal with common epidemics of his day, such as cholera, malaria, pneumonia, smallpox, diphtheria, and tuberculosis. Three of his children died from spinal meningitis and he became increasingly disillusioned with medical practices of his day. Because of this, in 1872, he established the healing art of osteopathy.[2]

A.T. Still became a wandering physician because his new ideas were not accepted in Kansas. He traveled throughout Kansas and Missouri, treated patients, and described his methods to countless people. For many years, Kirksville, Missouri

[a] Department of Family Medicine, University of Wisconsin School of Medicine and Public Health, 1100 Dela Plaine Court, Madison, WI 53715, USA
[b] Department of Family Medicine, University of Wisconsin School of Medicine and Public Health, 425 Wind Ridge Drive, Wausau, WI 54401, USA
* Corresponding author.
E-mail address: brian.earley@fammed.wisc.edu (B.E. Earley).

Prim Care Clin Office Pract 37 (2010) 49–64
doi:10.1016/j.pop.2009.09.001   **primarycare.theclinics.com**

was Dr Still's base while he traveled. By 1889, however, there were a great number of patients traveling to see Dr Still at his newly founded infirmary there. He no longer had to travel to practice osteopathic medicine. His practice grew, and he gained more respect.[2]

In 1892, Dr Still opened the American School of Osteopathy (ASO) in Kirksville, Missouri. He taught the art of osteopathic medicine through lecture, demonstration, and direct patient care. The first diplomas were awarded to 18 graduates of the ASO in 1894. Additional schools opened as osteopathic medicine began to spread throughout the United States.[2]

In the United States, *osteopathic medicine* has replaced the term *osteopathy* and *osteopathic physician* has replaced the term *osteopath*. The word "osteopath" now describes only practitioners before 1960. "Osteopathy" is the profession as practiced outside the United States (by practitioners who did not train at American Osteopathic Association [AOA]-accredited osteopathic medical colleges).[2]

EDUCATION, LICENSING, AND PRACTICE

As of May 2009, there are 25 osteopathic medical schools with 31 locations in 22 states.[3] Each school is accredited by the AOA's Commission on Osteopathic College Accreditation, which is recognized by the U.S. Department of Education.[4] Facts about osteopathic physicians are found in **Box 1**.

Application requirements for osteopathic and allopathic medical colleges are similar. Historically, osteopathic schools have placed increased emphasis on the interview to assess interpersonal communication skills.[4]

The curriculum at osteopathic medical schools involves 4 years of academic study, the same as in allopathic medical schools. The colleges of osteopathic medicine (COMs) emphasize preventive medicine and comprehensive patient care. Throughout the curriculum, students learn to use osteopathic principles and manipulative techniques to diagnose and treat patients. An additional 150 to 200 hours during medical school is spent learning osteopathic manipulative medicine (OMM).[7] After graduation, DOs complete residency training just as MDs do.[4] DOs can choose to complete an osteopathic, allopathic, or a dually accredited residency.

A study by Peters and colleagues[8] demonstrated that careers in primary care are better supported in osteopathic medical schools than in allopathic schools. Primary care is emphasized at osteopathic schools, and students are encouraged to pursue primary care careers by their faculty. Osteopathic medical schools also have a higher percentage of primary care faculty than do allopathic schools.

Box 1
Facts about osteopathic physicians

By the year 2020, there will be an estimated 100,000 practicing osteopathic physicians in the United States.

Approximately 65% of practicing DOs specialize in primary care.

DOs comprise 6% of the US physician population.

Many DOs practice in rural and other medically underserved communities.[4]

Approximately 70% of Family Medicine DOs use OMT, but less than 10 % use it during more than half of their patient encounters.[5]

Approximately 50% of all osteopathic physicians use OMT.[6]

Data from Refs.[4–6]

DOs must pass similar examinations as MDs to obtain state licensure. DOs can become board certified through allopathic licensure, osteopathic licensure, or both, depending on the type of residency completed. Through this licensure, osteopathic and allopathic physicians are the only 2 types of medical professionals who can obtain full medical practice rights.[4]

TENETS OF OSTEOPATHY

The basic concept of osteopathic medicine can be summarized with the first paragraph of the Kirksville consensus declaration, written in 1953:

Osteopathy, or Osteopathic Medicine, is a philosophy, a science and an art. Its philosophy embraces the concept of the unity of body structure and function in health and disease. Its science includes the chemical, physical and biological sciences related to the maintenance of health and the prevention, cure and alleviation of disease. Its art is the application of the philosophy and the science in the practice of osteopathic medicine and surgery in all its branches and specialties.[9]

The consensus declaration can be summarized into the 4 tenets of osteopathic medicine (**Box 2**).

SOMATIC DYSFUNCTION

The osteopathic physician must first identify improperly functioning and unbalanced lesions in a patient's musculoskeletal system. The most appropriate osteopathic term for these lesions is "somatic dysfunction" (**Box 3**). The osteopathic physician identifies areas of somatic dysfunction through palpation, distinguishing tender spots, asymmetric bony landmarks, restricted joint motion, and/or abnormal tissue texture. Tissue texture changes include temperature change, swelling, hyperesthesia, and/or firmness.

OSTEOPATHIC TECHNIQUES

Early in the profession, Dr Still taught students to use their knowledge of anatomy and physiology and clinical experience to best treat each patient instead of emphasizing specific techniques.[10] Because of this, various types of techniques have been developed (**Box 4**). High-velocity thrust techniques are recognized by many patients. Other techniques, however, focus on a more gentle correction of somatic dysfunction. These techniques may be more appropriate in acute injuries or disease processes and for hospitalized patients.

Box 2
Tenets of osteopathic medicine

1. The body is a unit.
2. The body possesses self-regulatory mechanisms.
3. Structure and function are reciprocally interrelated.
4. Rational treatment is based on an understanding of body unity, self-regulatory mechanisms, and the interrelationship of structure and function.

Data from Ward RC, Hruby RJ. Foundations for osteopathic medicine. 2nd edition. Philadelphia: Lippincott Williams & Wilkins; 2003.

Box 3
Somatic dysfunction

Impaired or altered function of related components of the somatic (body framework) system: skeletal, arthrodial, and myofascial structures and related vascular, lymphatic, and neural elements.[9]

Data from Ward RC, Hruby RJ. Foundations for osteopathic medicine. 2nd edition. Philadelphia: Lippincott Williams & Wilkins; 2003.

The decision to use one technique over another may depend on acuity of pain,[11,12] anxiety,[11] physician preference,[12] or potential contraindications. After every treatment, the osteopathic physician rechecks the structures to assess for correction. Osteopathic physicians use OMT not only to cure disease but also to put the patient's body in the best position to heal itself.

RISKS

OMT is quite safe. High-velocity techniques have the most potential risk because of the rapid "thrust." Most research, therefore, has been done on the safety of these

---

Box 4
Examples of various osteopathic manipulative techniques

High-velocity low-amplitude (HVLA) techniques: the physician uses a HVLA thrust to push through a joint restriction to restore the range of motion (ROM) of that joint.

Springing techniques: the physician repetitively, gently rocks or pulses against the restriction of a joint to restore the ROM of that joint.

Muscle energy techniques: the physician asks the patient to pull against the physician's resistance to rebalance the muscles around a dysfunctional joint.

Soft tissue techniques: the physician kneads, stretches, or applies inhibitory pressure to relax the soft tissues.[11]

Functional techniques: the physician monitors the soft tissues while small motions are applied to the joint to decrease resistance. These techniques often use the patient's breathing to cause the restriction in the joint to "release."

Strain-counterstrain techniques: these techniques involve palpating tender points and putting the joint in a position to take away the palpatory pain of these points. This position is held until the restriction releases (approximately 90 seconds).[9,12]

Facilitated positional release: in these techniques, the joint or tissue is taken to the position of most comfort. Traction or compression is applied to facilitate an immediate release of the tissue tension.

Still technique: a technique, thought to be developed by Dr Still, which is set up like facilitated positional release, but after traction or compression is applied, the joint is moved through it's restrictive barrier and then returned to neutral.

Cranial osteopathy: this gentle, manual technique emphasizes balancing the tensions of the dura.

Lymphatic techniques: various techniques that generally involve gentle techniques aimed at promoting the movement of the lymphatic fluid are used to promote healing from a number of conditions.

Data from Ward RC, Hruby RJ. Foundations for osteopathic medicine. 2nd edition. Philadelphia: Lippincott Williams & Wilkins; 2003; and Tettambel MA. Osteopathic treatment considerations for rheumatic diseases. J Am Osteopath Assoc 2001;101:18–20.

---

techniques. Most studies on the risks of spinal manipulation do not differentiate between manipulation done by chiropractors, therapists, osteopathic physicians, or other practitioners. Therefore, the data included here relate to spinal manipulation done by any practitioner, unless noted otherwise. To distinguish between common, mild reactions and rare, more severe side effects, Gibbons and Tehan[13] described a classification of adverse reactions including (1) transient, (2) substantive reversible impairment, and (3) serious nonreversible impairment.

Common transient effects include local pain, headache, tiredness or fatigue, and radiating pain.[13,14] Transient effects occur in 30% to 61% of patients, begin within 4 hours after spinal manipulation, and usually resolve within 24 hours.[13,14]

Substantive reversible impairment includes disk herniation, nerve root compression, and fracture. Worsening disk problems are the most common of these because of the frequent association between back pain and disk disease. One systematic review found that worsening disk disease in patients with lumbar disk herniation occurs less often than 1 in 3.7 million patients.[13] It is unknown whether this progression would have occurred without manipulation.[13] Manipulation is relatively contraindicated in patients with signs or symptoms of herniated disk or with acute midline back pain until fracture or herniated disk have been ruled out radiographically.[15]

Most attention has been paid to serious nonreversible risks. The most common of these is iatrogenic stroke. The reported incidence of stroke varies from 1 in 10,000 to 1 in 5.85 million cervical manipulations. Rarely, vertebral dissection can also occur with manipulation of the neck. Because of the spontaneous nature of this disease, however, it is unknown whether manipulation actually causes vertebral dissection.[13,16] In a review of injuries caused by manipulative treatments between 1925 and 1993, only 185 cases of serious injury were reported, and only 2 of these involved DOs.[17] Thirty-six patients had been treated by an untrained professional.[17]

Most adverse effects of spinal manipulation are associated with

1. Misdiagnosis (tumors or metastasis) causing delay in treatment
2. Coagulation dyscrasia (causing meningeal hematoma)
3. Cervical manipulation
4. Disk herniation
5. Improper technique by untrained personnel.[18]

Keys to safety include appropriate training, skill refinement through regular practice, and a thorough history and physical examination.[17] Manipulation seems to be significantly safer than other modalities (including antiinflammatory medications)[16] commonly used for musculoskeletal conditions.[16] Finally, OMT seems to be safe in the pediatric population also.[12]

RESEARCH

Before looking at OMT research for different conditions, several questions should be discussed.

Can Osteopathic Research Fit in the Allopathic Research Model?

Double-blind manipulation studies are difficult because the DO cannot be masked to treatment. Some argue that conventional clinical "reductionist" research, reducing treatment into components to randomize 1 component, cannot adequately investigate holistic treatments.[19,20] The osteopathic physician places the patient at the heart of the holistic healing process, making it difficult to separate the components of treatment into pieces that can be studied.[19]

How Does One Do Sham Manipulation?

Single-blinded studies including sham manipulation also raise some concerns. Sham treatments should be ineffective, but must seem plausible to patients.[21] Different types of sham manipulation include palpatory diagnostic procedures, "massage" techniques, light touch, or inactive instruments. Some of these studies prove blinding effectiveness.[21] The more similarly sham manipulation mimics OMT, the more it positively acts on the body, making it no longer "sham." Sham manipulation may work better on patients who are naive to manipulation and when "gentle treatment techniques" are used, because the treatment mimics the "light touch" of sham treatment.[21] The use of placebo control in studies remains one of the most controversial subjects in osteopathic research.[22]

Are Studies Done on Chiropractic Manipulation Valid in Osteopathic Medicine?

Physical therapy, massage therapy, chiropractic manipulation, and osteopathy all incorporate types of manual medicine. There are more chiropractic than osteopathic research studies. Many researchers assume that chiropractic findings cross over to osteopathic practice. However, most chiropractic research involves only high-velocity short-lever adjustments, whereas DOs use many types of manipulation. Osteopathic physicians also practice manipulation as an adjuvant to traditional management of conditions,[23] whereas chiropractors do not offer traditional medical management.[23]

Two chiropractic studies that exemplified the problem of interchanging chiropractic findings to osteopathic practice were examined by Mein and colleagues.[24] In each study, the treatment group and sham manipulation group showed significant improvement over the control group but little difference between each other. Therefore, manipulation was concluded to be ineffective for both. On further evaluation, however, the sham manipulation was similar to osteopathic or other manual medicine treatments.[24] Therefore, each study actually showed similar effectiveness between 2 different types of manual treatments.

Has Enough Emphasis Been Put on Osteopathic Research?

Traditionally, research has not been a significant component of the osteopathic profession.[25] However, due to an increased emphasis on research by the AOA, between 1989 and 1999, there was a 37% increase in extramurally funded research at COMs over these years.[25] However, 74% of this research was done in basic biomedical science.[25] Of the 189 research projects that were funded by the National Institutes of Health (NIH) Office of Alternative Medicine between 1993 and 1999, none went to a COM.[25] In 1999, research represented 26% of expenditures at publicly assisted allopathic schools compared with only 7% at public osteopathic schools (32% vs 2% at private schools).[26]

What is the Future of Osteopathic Research?

Further emphases on clinical research in the late 1990s led the profession to establish the Osteopathic Research Center to improve research on OMT.[27] The profession invested $1.1 million into this center. By the end of 2005 the center had generated $8.6 million in research funding.[27] Grants won by researchers at COMs increased from $26.8 million in 1999 to $101.7 million in 2004 (380% increase).[27] The amount awarded to DOs increased from $4.4 million to $12.6 million (280% increase). Between 1999 and 2004, money awarded by the NIH to the COMs tripled, and 3 research grants, totaling more than $3.2 million, became the first OMM studies to be awarded NIH grants.[27]

The profession's emphasis on research needs to continue to grow. Improved research curricula at osteopathic medical schools,[28] larger blinded studies,[29] larger studies on the cost-effectiveness of manipulation,[30,31] and more collaborative groups of experienced osteopathic researchers working together[32] have been proposed to improve research within the profession. Norman Gevitz stated in an article in the March 2001 issue of *The Journal of the American Osteopathic Association*:

> For osteopathic medicine to move forward, it must be evidence-based. The studies that can provide this evidentiary foundation can only come from within the profession. It is the absolute responsibility of this profession to provide the researchers and resources to accomplish this goal, and as a result, ensure the future of osteopathic medicine.[33]

Even with recent research progress, these words are as true today as they were in 2001.

MANIPULATION FOR CONDITIONS
Low Back Pain

Low back pain is the most common condition cited by patients seeing a DO, accounting for approximately 11% of visits to DOs,[34] which explains why it is also the most commonly studied condition (**Table 1**). Because of an osteopathic physician's use of traditional and complementary therapy, they avoid costs incurred in sending patients to separate manual medicine professionals. Osteopathic physicians treat back pain with fewer visits than chiropractors. In comparison to allopathic physicians, DOs make fewer referrals, admit a lower percentage of patients to the hospital, order fewer radiographs, and prescribe less medication for patients with back pain.[35]

A meta-analysis of randomized controlled studies done by Licciardone and colleagues[35] in 2005 evaluated the literature for OMT used for acute low back pain. Six randomized controlled studies (3 from the United States and 3 from the United Kingdom), from 1973 to 2001, were reviewed, and they included a total of 525 patients with low back pain treated by osteopathic physicians. The investigators concluded that "OMT significantly reduces low back pain" in the acute setting ($P<.01$) with short term ($P = .01$), intermediate-term ($P<.001$), and long-term ($P = .03$) follow-ups.[35]

Further evaluation of low back pain manipulation studies shows that OMT

- decreases use of medications (analgesics, antiinflammatory agents, and muscle relaxants) and physical therapy[36]
- improves physical and psychological outcomes with little additional cost[37]
- is more effective for acute than chronic low back pain.[38]

Other Musculoskeletal Conditions
Neck pain

Manipulation of the cervical spine is another common use of OMT. However, there are few randomized controlled trials on the benefits of OMT for acute neck pain. A recent study randomized 58 patients with less than 3 weeks of neck pain into 2 groups. One group was treated with OMT and the other was treated with ketorolac 30 mg intramuscularly without placebo control. Both groups showed a significant reduction in pain intensity ($P<.001$), but the OMT group showed a significantly greater decrease in pain intensity ($P = .02$).[39]

Table 1
Patient-oriented practice recommendations

Clinical Recommendation	Evidence Rating	References
OMT significantly reduces acute low back pain with effects lasting up to 3 months	A	35
OMT significantly improves neck pain immediately after it is performed on a patient with acute neck pain and when compared with injection of ketorolac 30 mg intramuscularly	B	39
OMT immediately improves ankle edema and pain in patients with acute first- or second-degree ankle sprains and significantly improves ankle ROM 1 week after it is performed on patients with acute ankle sprains	B	40
OMT combined with standard medical care for fibromyalgia is more efficacious than treatment of fibromyalgia with standard medical care alone	B	41
OMT decreases acute headache in patients with a history of chronic tension-type headaches	B	43
Weekly OMT increases number of headache-free days and headache diary rating (combination of headache frequency and intensity) in patients with chronic tension-type headaches	B	44
OMT significantly reduces hospital stay and length of intravenous antibiotic requirements in elderly patients hospitalized with pneumonia when added to traditional pneumonia treatment	B	45,46
OMT appears to be as effective as incentive spirometry at preventing postoperative atelectasis after cholecystectomy and causes quicker return to preoperative values for FVC and FEV_1 than incentive spirometry	B	48
Patients in labor with low back pain who receive OMT require less narcotic medication than those not treated with OMT	B	53
Patients who receive OMT during pregnancy are less likely to have meconium-stained amniotic fluid on delivery and are less likely to have preterm delivery	B	52
OMT significantly reduces multiple menopausal symptoms including hot flashes and night sweats in symptomatic patients with effects lasting at least 5 weeks after treatment	B	54
Cranial manipulation significantly reduces crying and increases the time spent sleeping in infants diagnosed with colic	B	56
OMT added to standard care in pediatric patients with recurrent otitis media significantly reduces episodes of AOM, insertion of ventilatory tubes, and mean surgery-free months	B	57
OMT provided to hospitalized patients with pancreatitis significantly reduces the number of days in the hospital for those patients	B	59
OMT performed on patients with Parkinson disease significantly improves stride length, cadence, and maximum velocities of various joints acutely	B	60

Ankle sprain
Another study randomized 55 adults who presented to an emergency department with a unilateral first- or second-degree acute ankle sprain. One group received OMT and the other group received standard care for acute ankle injuries. No placebo treatment was attempted. Patients were evaluated for edema, ROM, and pain immediately after manipulation and at a 1-week follow-up appointment. Improvements were significant acutely in the OMT group for edema ($P<.001$) and pain ($P<.001$). At the follow-up visit, changes in ROM ($P = .01$) were significant. Long-term follow-up was not studied.[40]

Fibromyalgia
The effect of OMT on fibromyalgia was studied by randomizing 24 female patients into 4 groups: (1) OMT, (2) OMT and teaching (patients were taught home tender point treatment), (3) moist heat, and (4) no additional treatment. Patients were allowed to continue their chronic medications. Significant findings favoring OMT were found in measures of pain threshold, perceived pain, attitude toward treatment, activities of daily living, and chronic pain, although P values were not reported for each individual measure. The study was described as "placebo-controlled" but placebo manipulation was not described.[41]

Postoperative: OMT after knee and hip arthroplasty
OMT has not been found to be effective for rehabilitation after orthopedic surgery. Although 2 previous studies showed improvements in the OMT groups, a more recent randomized placebo-controlled study did not. This study evaluated 60 patients in a rehabilitation unit after having knee or hip arthroplasty. The only significant difference was decreased rehabilitation efficiency in the group treated with OMT ($P = .01$) and a trend toward increased length of stay. With these negative outcomes, the investigators did not believe that a larger study was likely to show significant improvements in the OMT group.[42]

Headaches

Acute tension-type headaches
OMT has also been studied for use in patients with tension-type headaches secondary to associated muscle tension in the neck. A small randomized controlled study evaluated the effect of OMT on acute headaches in patients with chronic tension-type headaches. Twenty-two patients were divided into 3 groups: (1) OMT, (2) palpatory diagnosis (placebo), or (3) 10 minutes of relaxation (control). The group of patients treated with OMT showed significant decrease in rated headache pain ($P<.0003$).[43]

Chronic tension-type headaches
OMT for chronic tension-type headaches was studied in 2006. Twenty-nine patients were randomized into either an OMT group or control group without placebo control. Both groups did regular home relaxation exercises and continued chronic medications. One group received 3 osteopathic treatments (once weekly). Significant improvement was shown for the treatment group in the number of headache-free days ($P = .016$), in a trend toward improved overall severity of headaches ($P = .075$), and in headache diary rating (combination of headache frequency and intensity, $P = .059$).[44]

Respiratory Conditions

Pneumonia (hospitalized patients)
OMT has also been studied in several respiratory illnesses. Positive results were shown in a small randomized controlled study on using OMT in elderly, hospitalized

patients with pneumonia[45]; therefore, a larger study was conducted. Fifty-eight patients were randomized into a treatment group receiving standardized OMT or a placebo treatment of light touch. The duration of intravenous antibiotic use was almost 2 days shorter in the treatment group than in the control group ($P = .005$). The hospital stay was also 2 days shorter in the treatment group than in the control group ($P = .014$).[46] Because of the results of these previous studies, a 5-site, hospital-based, prospective, randomized controlled trial to evaluate the efficacy of OMT as an adjuvant treatment for elderly patients hospitalized with pneumonia has been completed. The results have yet to be reported.[47]

Postoperative atelectasis

In another inpatient study, 42 patients were randomized to treatment with OMT or incentive spirometry to prevent postoperative atelectasis after cholecystectomy. Rates of atelectasis were the same for both groups, but the OMT group had a quicker return to preoperative values for forced vital capacity (FVC) and forced expiratory volume in 1 second (FEV_1) ($P<.01$).[48]

Asthma

Additional OMT studies have been conducted on asthma in adults and children.[49,50] However, no osteopathic studies were included in the most recent Cochrane Review on the subject because neither of the osteopathic studies observed the patient at least 2 weeks after the manipulation (part of the inclusion criteria).[51] There is a definite need for better studies to be done to assess the effect of OMT on this disease.

Obstetrics and Gynecology

OMT has historically been used during pregnancy, but few studies have been done on applications and outcomes.[52] Studies in the early twentieth century showed decreased labor times, decreased forceps deliveries, and decreased maternal death.[52]

Back pain during labor

In 1982, a retrospective study on laboring women with lumbar pain was conducted. Those who were treated with OMT during labor had less use of narcotic medication when compared with those who did not ($P<.01$) or those who received thoracic OMT as a placebo treatment ($P<.05$). Lumbar OMT did not affect length of labor in this study.[53]

OMT done during pregnancy

A more recent retrospective study of pregnant patients treated with multiple episodes of OMT during pregnancy compared 160 women who received OMT throughout pregnancy to 161 women who did not. The study demonstrated decreased frequency of meconium-stained amniotic fluid ($P<.001$) and decreased occurrence of preterm delivery ($P<.01$). A marginally significant decrease in the use of forceps ($P = .07$) was also shown.[52]

A gynecologic study randomized 30 women experiencing menopausal symptoms into manipulation versus placebo groups. This study showed a greater reduction of hot flashes ($P = .016$), night sweats ($P = .021$), urinary frequency ($P = .021$), and depression ($P = .042$) in the treatment group during the 10 weeks of the study. Improvements remained similar for hot flashes ($P = .007$) and night sweats ($P = .016$), and improvement in insomnia ($P = .018$) became significant 5 weeks after treatment. Testosterone levels were significantly lowered in the treatment group ($P = .028$) but did not change in the control group.[54]

Finally, a small randomized study with only 12 patients was done on dysmenorrheal subjects with low back pain. Two patients received OMT, 2 received no OMT or placebo, and 8 received OMT during 1 menstrual cycle but did not receive OMT during the next. All subjects treated with OMT claimed improvement of their back pain.[55]

Pediatric Conditions

Infantile colic
OMT is commonly used in conditions that do not have effective traditional treatments, including infantile colic. One study randomized 28 infants with colic into 2 groups to receive either osteopathic cranial manipulation or no treatment. The study showed a highly significant improvement in time spent crying ($P<.001$) and time spent sleeping ($P<.002$).[56]

Otitis media
In a study on the effects of OMT on pediatric patients with multiple episodes of acute otitis media (AOM), patients were randomized into a group receiving either OMT and routine care or routine care alone (without placebo). The group receiving OMM had less episodes of AOM ($P = .04$), fewer surgical procedures ($P = .03$), and more mean surgery-free months ($P = .01$). There was an increased number of normal tympanograms in the intervention groups ($P = .02$).[57]

Given the safety of manipulative treatments in children, the presence of pediatric conditions without other effective medical therapy, and the increased emphasis on decreasing medication use by children, more research using OMT in other pediatric conditions seems appropriate.

Other Conditions

Depression
OMT has shown a positive effect in several other conditions. In a small randomized controlled study of 17 patients with depression, a group treated with OMT, paroxetine, and psychotherapy had more improved depression scores by week 8 than those receiving placebo (with structural examination), paroxetine, and psychotherapy. Significance of results was not reported and dropout rate was high.[58]

Pancreatitis
A study on the effects of OMT in patients hospitalized with pancreatitis randomized 14 patients to receive OMT with standard care or standard care alone. Patients in the treatment group spent significantly fewer days in the hospital before discharge (mean reduction of 3.5 days, $P = .039$). However, there were no significant differences in time to food intake or in use of pain medication between the 2 groups.[59]

Parkinson disease
A small (20 patients) randomized study with placebo control looked at gait changes in patients with Parkinson disease. Patients receiving sham manipulation of limb ROM evaluation and structural measurements showed no significant change with treatment compared with their baseline. Significant changes including stride length, cadence, and maximum velocities of various joints, however, were shown in the OMT treatment group, who each received a standard 14 osteopathic techniques.[60]

SUMMARY

Osteopathic medicine is defined as "A complete system of medical care with philosophy that combines the needs of the patient with current practice of medicine, surgery and obstetrics. [It] emphasizes the interrelationship between structure and function, and has an appreciation of the body's ability to heal itself."[61] It is within this philosophy that the osteopathic physician uses OMT to place the patient's body in the best position to heal itself. Therefore it serves as a helpful complement to allopathic traditional care for several common conditions (**Box 5**).

Box 5
Incorporating OMT into an allopathic practice

How to find a DO near you: http://www.osteopathic.org/directory.cfm

State and regional osteopathic organizations: http://www.osteopathic.org/index.cfm?au=A&;PageID=lcl_assoc

Osteopathic medical schools: http://www.aacom.org (Web site for the American Association of Colleges of Osteopathic Medicine)

General osteopathic information (American Osteopathic Association)

    http://www.osteopathic.org (general public)

    http://www.do-online.org (health care professionals)

Common conditions treated with OMT[5]

  1. Back pain

    a. Sprains, strains, and spasm of all areas of the back and neck

  2. Other joint pain

  3. Headaches

  4. Sinusitis

  5. Upper respiratory infection

  6. Fibromyalgia

  7. Asthma

  8. Carpal tunnel

  9. Pneumonia

  10. Chronic obstructive pulmonary disease

  11. Sciatica

  12. Pelvic pain

  13. Bronchitis

  14. Temporomandibular joint disorder

  15. Pregnancy

  16. Radiculopathy

  17. Arthritis

Number of sessions of OMT needed:

The number and frequency of sessions used by an osteopathic physician varies depending on the type of condition, chronicity of the condition, the patient's response to previous OMT, and other factors. In general, acute conditions require fewer sessions of OMT and patients frequently have significant improvement with as little as 1 treatment. Chronic conditions often need more sessions of OMT, but generally these treatments become less frequent as the chronic condition improves.

There are risks to osteopathic medicine as there are with any medical treatment. Transient effects including local pain, headache, tiredness or fatigue, and radiating pain are common but resolve quickly. Substantive reversible impairment and serious nonreversible risks are much less common. These risks include disk herniation, nerve root compression, fracture, iatrogenic stroke, and vertebral dissection. Patients at risk for these conditions should have appropriate workup done, before the manipulation is performed.

Research has not traditionally been a significant component of the osteopathic profession, but the profession is trying to change this. Significant improvement has been achieved in the last 25 years in the amount and quality of osteopathic research. There are limitations to research of OMT, because these studies cannot be blinded to the physician and sham manipulation is difficult.

This article has outlined many of the available randomized studies that have researched OMT for different medical conditions. Manipulation done by other health care professionals was not included, because it cannot be assumed that findings from research done by these other professions crosses over to osteopathic manipulation.

Good research has been done showing the effectiveness of OMT for low back pain. OMT seems to be effective for other musculoskeletal conditions, including cervical pain, acute ankle pain, and fibromyalgia, and for certain types of headaches. Various types of respiratory applications, including pneumonia, prevention of postoperative atelectasis, and asthma, have been studied with good results. OMT seems to benefit pregnant patients and patients with dysmenorrheal and menopausal symptoms. Pediatric patients with colic seem to improve after OMT and children with history of multiple episodes of otitis media improve after OMT. Finally, OMT has shown effectiveness in depression, in patients hospitalized with pancreatitis, and in patients with Parkinson disease.

The osteopathic profession is a unique blend of traditional and complementary treatments that is beneficial for the health care consumer.

ACKNOWLEDGMENTS

We would like to thank Christopher Hooper-Lane, MLS, AHIP for his contributions to the literature search. We would also like to thank Bret Ripley, DO and Jerri Ustby-Cruz-Bye for their review of the article and recommendations about the content.

REFERENCES

1. Osteopathic medical profession report. Available at: http://www.osteopathic.org/index.cfm?PageID=aoa_ompreport_profession. Accessed May 15, 2009.
2. Andrew Taylor still establishes osteopathy. Available at: http://history.osteopathic.org/osteopathy.shtml. Accessed May 3, 2009.
3. Member colleges. Available at: http://www.aacom.org/people/colleges/Pages/default.aspx. Accessed May 3, 2009.
4. Osteopathic medicine. Available at: http://www.osteopathic.org/index.cfm?PageID=ost_omed. Accessed May 3, 2009.
5. Johnson S, Kurtz M, Kurtz J. Variables influencing the use of osteopathic manipulative treatment in family practice. J Am Osteopath Assoc 1997;97:80–7.
6. Spaeth D, Pheley A. Use of osteopathic manipulative treatment by Ohio osteopathic physicians in various specialties. J Am Osteopath Assoc 2003;103:16–26.
7. Johnson KH, Raczek JA, Meyer D. Integrating osteopathic training into family practice residencies. Fam Med 1998;30:345–9.

8. Peters AS, Clark-Chiarelli N, Block SD. Comparison of osteopathic and allopathic medical schools' support for primary care. J Gen Intern Med 1999;14:730–9.

9. Ward RC, Hruby RJ. Foundations for osteopathic medicine. 2nd edition. Philadelphia: Lippincott Williams & Wilkins; 2003.

10. Chikly BJ. Manual techniques addressing the lymphatic system: origins and development. J Am Osteopath Assoc 2005;105:457–64.

11. Tettambel MA. Osteopathic treatment considerations for rheumatic diseases. J Am Osteopath Assoc 2001;101:18–20.

12. Hayes NM, Bezilla TA. Incidence of iatrogenesis associated with osteopathic manipulative treatment of pediatric patients. J Am Osteopath Assoc 2006;106:605.

13. Gibbons P, Tehan P. HVLA thrust techniques: what are the risks? Int J Osteopath Med 2006;9:4–12.

14. Senstad O, Leboeuf-Yde C, Borchgrevink C. Frequency and characteristics of side effects of spinal manipulative therapy. Spine 1997;22:435–41.

15. Powell FC, Hanigan WC, Olivero WC. A risk/benefit analysis of spinal manipulation therapy for relief of lumbar or cervical pain. Neurosurgery 1993;33:73–8.

16. Stevinson C, Ernst E. Risks associated with spinal manipulation. Am J Med 2002; 112:566–71.

17. Vick D, McKay C, Zengerle C. The safety of manipulative treatment: review of the literature from 1925 to 1993. J Am Osteopath Assoc 1996;96:113–5.

18. Shekelle P, Coulter I. Cervical spine manipulation: summary report of a systematic review of the literature and a multidisciplinary expert panel. J Spinal Disord 1997; 10:223–8.

19. Patterson MM. Research in OMT: what is the question and do we understand it? J Am Osteopath Assoc 2007;107:8.

20. Korr IM. Osteopathic research: the needed paradigm shift. J Am Osteopath Assoc 1991;91(156):161–8, 170–1.

21. Noll DR, Degenhardt BF, Stuart M, et al. Effectiveness of a sham protocol and adverse effects in a clinical trial of osteopathic manipulative treatment in nursing home patients. J Am Osteopath Assoc 2004;104:107–13.

22. Licciardone JC, Russo DP. Blinding protocols, treatment credibility, and expectancy: methodologic issues in clinical trials of osteopathic manipulative treatment. J Am Osteopath Assoc 2006;106:457–63.

23. Friedman H. Osteopathy vs chiropractic. J Fam Pract 1993;37:221–2.

24. Mein E, Greenman P, McMillin D, et al. Manual medicine diversity: research pitfalls and the emerging medical paradigm. J Am Osteopath Assoc 2001;101: 441–4.

25. Guillory V, Sharp G. Research at US colleges of osteopathic medicine: a decade of growth. J Am Osteopath Assoc 2003;103:176–81.

26. Rodgers F, Dyer M. Adopting research. J Am Osteopath Assoc 2000;100:234–7.

27. Clearfield MB, Smith-Barbaro P, Guillory VJ, et al. Research funding at colleges of osteopathic medicine: 15 years of growth. J Am Osteopath Assoc 2007;107:469.

28. Licciardone JC. Educating osteopaths to be researchers–what role should research methods and statistics have in an undergraduate curriculum? Int J Osteopath Med 2008;11:62–8.

29. Cardarelli R. Recurring limitations in OMT research. J Am Osteopath Assoc 2006; 106:112–3.

30. Williams NH, Edwards RT, Linck P, et al. Cost-utility analysis of osteopathy in primary care: results from a pragmatic randomized controlled trial. Fam Pract 2004;21:643–50.

31. Gamber R, Holland S, Russo DP, et al. Cost-effective osteopathic manipulative medicine: a literature review of cost-effectiveness analyses for osteopathic manipulative treatment. J Am Osteopath Assoc 2005;105:357–67.
32. Lucas NP, Moran RW. Researching osteopathy: who is responsible? Int J Osteopath Med 2007;10:33–5.
33. Gevitz N. Researched and demonstrated: inquiry and infrastructure at osteopathic institutions. J Am Osteopath Assoc 2001;101:174–9.
34. Cypress B. Characteristics of physician visits for back symptoms: a national perspective. Am J Public Health 1983;73:389–95.
35. Licciardone JC, Brimhall AK, King LN. Osteopathic manipulative treatment for low back pain: a systematic review and meta-analysis of randomized controlled trials. BMC Musculoskelet Disord 2005;6:43.
36. Andersson GBJ, Lucente T, Davis AM, et al. A comparison of osteopathic spinal manipulation with standard care for patients with low back pain. N Engl J Med 1999;341:1426–31.
37. Williams NH, Wilkinson C, Russell I, et al. Randomized osteopathic manipulation study (ROMANS): pragmatic trial for spinal pain in primary care. Fam Pract 2003; 20:662–9.
38. Licciardone JC, Stoll ST, Fulda KG, et al. Osteopathic manipulative treatment for chronic low back pain: a randomized controlled trial. Spine 2003;28:1355.
39. McReynolds TM, Sheridan BJ. Intramuscular ketorolac versus osteopathic manipulative treatment in the management of acute neck pain in the emergency department: a randomized clinical trial. J Am Osteopath Assoc 2005;105:57–68.
40. Eisenhart A, Gaeta T, Yens D. Osteopathic manipulative treatment in the emergency department for patients with acute ankle injuries. J Am Osteopath Assoc 2003;103:417–21.
41. Gamber R, Shores J, Russo D, et al. Osteopathic manipulative treatment in conjunction with medication relieves pain associated with fibromyalgia syndrome: results of a randomized clinical pilot project. J Am Osteopath Assoc 2002;102:321–5.
42. Licciardone JC, Stoll ST, Cardarelli KM, et al. A randomized controlled trial of osteopathic manipulative treatment following knee or hip arthroplasty. J Am Osteopath Assoc 2004;104:193–202.
43. Hoyt W, Shaffer F, Bard D, et al. Osteopathic manipulation in the treatment of muscle-contraction headache. J Am Osteopath Assoc 1979;78:322–5.
44. Anderson RE, Seniscal C. A comparison of selected osteopathic treatment and relaxation for tension-type headaches. Headache 2006;46:1273–80.
45. Noll D, Shores J, Bryman P, et al. Adjunctive osteopathic manipulative treatment in the elderly hospitalized with pneumonia: a pilot study. J Am Osteopath Assoc 1999;99:143–6.
46. Noll D, Shores J, Gamber R, et al. Benefits of osteopathic manipulative treatment for hospitalized elderly patients with pneumonia. J Am Osteopath Assoc 2000; 100:776–82.
47. Noll DR, Degenhardt BF, Fossum C, et al. Clinical and research protocol for osteopathic manipulative treatment of elderly patients with pneumonia. J Am Osteopath Assoc 2008;108:508.
48. Sleszynski S, Kelso A. Comparison of thoracic manipulation with incentive spirometry in preventing postoperative atelectasis. J Am Osteopath Assoc 1993;93:834–8.
49. Bockenhauer S, Julliard K, Lo K, et al. Quantifiable effects of osteopathic manipulative techniques on patients with chronic asthma. J Am Osteopath Assoc 2002; 102:371–5.

50. Guiney PA, Chou R, Vianna A, et al. Effects of osteopathic manipulative treatment on pediatric patients with asthma: a randomized controlled trial. J Am Osteopath Assoc 2005;105:7–12.

51. Hondras MA, Linde K, Jones AP. Manual therapy for asthma. Cochrane Database Syst Rev 2005;(2):CD001002.

52. King H, Tettambel M, Lockwood M, et al. Osteopathic manipulative treatment in prenatal care: a retrospective case control design study. J Am Osteopath Assoc 2003;103:577–82.

53. Guthrie RA, Martin RH. Effect of pressure applied to the upper thoracic (placebo) versus lumbar areas (osteopathic manipulative treatment) for inhibition of lumbar myalgia during labor. J Am Osteopath Assoc 1982;82:247–51.

54. Cleary C, Fox J. Menopausal symptoms: an osteopathic investigation. Complement Ther Med 1994;2:181–6.

55. Boesler D, Warner M, Alpers A, et al. Efficacy of high-velocity low-amplitude manipulative technique in subjects with low-back pain during menstrual cramping. J Am Osteopath Assoc 1993;93:203–8.

56. Hayden C, Mullinger B. A preliminary assessment of the impact of cranial osteopathy for the relief of infantile colic. Complement Ther Clin Pract 2006;12:83–90.

57. Mills MV, Henley CE, Barnes LLB, et al. The use of osteopathic manipulative treatment as adjuvant therapy in children with recurrent acute otitis media. Arch Pediatr Adolesc Med 2003;157:861–6.

58. Plotkin B, Rodos J, Kappler R, et al. Adjunctive osteopathic manipulative treatment in women with depression: a pilot study. J Am Osteopath Assoc 2001;101:517–23.

59. Radjieski J, Lumley M, Cantieri M. Effect of osteopathic manipulative treatment of length of stay for pancreatitis: a randomized pilot study. J Am Osteopath Assoc 1998;98:264–72.

60. Wells M, Giantinoto S, D'Agate D, et al. Standard osteopathic manipulative treatment acutely improves gait performance in patients with Parkinson's disease. J Am Osteopath Assoc 1999;99:92–8.

61. Glover J. Glossary of osteopathic terminology usage guide. Available at: http://www.osteopathic.org/pdf/sir_collegegloss.pdf. Accessed May 9, 2009.

Prolotherapy in Primary Care Practice

David Rabago, MD*, Andrew Slattengren, DO,
Aleksandra Zgierska, MD, PhD

KEYWORDS

- Prolotherapy • Injection therapy • Osteoarthritis
- Tendinopathy • Low back pain
- Chronic musculoskeletal pain

Prolotherapy is an injection-based complementary and alternative medical (CAM) therapy for chronic musculoskeletal pain. It has been used for approximately 100 years; however, its modern applications can be traced to the 1950s when the prolotherapy injection protocols were formalized by George Hackett,[1] a general surgeon in the United States, based on his clinical experience of more than 30 years. Prolotherapy techniques and injected solutions vary by condition, clinical severity, and practitioner preferences; a core principle is that a fairly small volume of an irritant or sclerosing solution is injected at sites on painful ligament and tendon insertions and in adjacent joint space over several treatment sessions.[1,2] Interest in prolotherapy among physicians and patients is high. It is becoming increasingly popular in the United States and internationally and is actively used in clinical practice.[3,4] A 1993 survey sent to osteopathic physicians estimated that 95 practitioners in the United States were estimated to have performed prolotherapy on approximately 450,000 patients. However, only 27% of surveys were returned; consequently, the true number of practitioners was probably dramatically underestimated.[5] No formal survey has been done since 1993. The current number of practitioners actively practicing prolotherapy is unknown but is probably several thousand in the United States based on attendance at continuing medical education (CME) conferences and physician listings on relevant Web sites. Prolotherapy has been assessed as a treatment for a wide variety of painful chronic musculoskeletal conditions that are refractory to "standard-of care" therapies. Although anecdotal clinical success guides the use of prolotherapy for many conditions, clinical trial literature supporting evidence-based

---

Grant Support: None.

Portions of this article were adapted from Rabago D, Best T, Beamsly M, Patterson J. A systematic review of prolotherapy for chronic musculoskeletal pain. Clin J Sports Med 2005;15(5):376–80; with permission.

Department of Family Medicine, University of Wisconsin School of Medicine and Public Health, 777 South Mills Street, Madison, WI 53715, USA

* Corresponding author.

E-mail address: David.rabago@fammed.wisc.edu (D. Rabago).

Prim Care Clin Office Pract 37 (2010) 65–80
doi:10.1016/j.pop.2009.09.013
0095-4543/10/$ – see front matter © 2010 Elsevier Inc. All rights reserved.

decision-making for the use of prolotherapy exists for low back pain (LBP), several tendinopathies, and osteoarthritis (OA).

The name of prolotherapy has changed over time. Consistent with existing hypotheses and understanding of possible mechanisms of action, the name of this therapy has evolved. Nomenclature has reflected practitioners' perceptions of prolotherapy's therapeutic effects on tissue. Historically, this injection therapy was called sclerotherapy because early solutions were thought to be scar-forming. Prolotherapy is currently the most commonly used name and is based on the presumed "proliferative" effects on chronically injured tissue. It has also been called regenerative injection therapy (RIT),[2,6] and some contemporary authors name the therapy according to the injected solution.[7] The precise mechanism of action is not known.

The National Institute of Health identifies prolotherapy as a CAM therapy and has funded 2 ongoing clinical prolotherapy trials. The Centers for Medicare and Medicaid Services and Veteran's Administration have reviewed the prolotherapy literature for LBP and all musculoskeletal indications and determined existing evidence to be inconclusive. Neither recommends third-party compensation for prolotherapy. However, their review did not include the most recent clinically positive studies or reviews.[7–9] Private insurers are beginning to cover prolotherapy for selected indications and clinical circumstances; however, most patients pay "out-of-pocket."

PROLOTHERAPY TECHNIQUE

Although no formal practice guidelines have been published, prolotherapy treatment commonly consists of several injection sessions delivered every 2 to 6 weeks over several months. During an individual prolotherapy session, therapeutic solutions are injected at sites of painful and tender ligament and tendon insertions and in adjacent joint spaces. Injected solutions ("proliferants") have historically been hypothesized to cause local irritation, with subsequent inflammation and tissue healing, resulting in enlargement and strengthening of damaged ligamentous, tendon, and intra-articular structures.[10,11] These processes were thought to improve joint stability, biomechanics, and function, and ultimately, to decrease pain.[1,2]

MECHANISM OF ACTION

The mechanism of action for prolotherapy has not been clearly established and, until recently, received little attention. Supported by pilot-level evidence, the 3 most commonly used prolotherapy solutions have been hypothesized to act via different pathways: hypertonic dextrose by osmotic rupture of local cells, phenol-glycerine-glucose (P2G) by local cellular irritation, and morrhuate sodium by chemotactic attraction of inflammatory mediators[12] and sclerosing of pathologic neovascularity associated with tendinopathy.[13,14] The potential of prolotherapy to stimulate release of growth factors favoring soft tissue healing has also been suggested as a possible mechanism.[15,16]

In vitro and animal model data have not fully corroborated these hypotheses. An inflammatory response in a rat knee ligament model has been reported for each solution, although it was not significantly different from that caused by needle stick alone or saline injections.[17] However, animal model data suggest a significant biologic effect of morrhuate sodium and dextrose solutions compared with controls. Rabbit medial collateral ligaments injected with morrhuate sodium were significantly stronger (31%), larger (47%), and thicker (28%), and had a larger collagen fiber diameter (56%) than saline-injected controls[10]; increase in cell number, water content, ground substance amount, and various inflammatory cell types were hypothesized to account for these changes.[11] Rat patellar tendons injected with morrhuate sodium were able to withstand a mean maximal load of 136% ($\pm$28%)—significantly more than the uninjected control tendon.[18] In the same study, tendons injected with saline control solution were significantly weaker than uninjected controls.[18] Dextrose has been minimally assessed in animal models. Recent studies showed that injured medial collateral rat ligaments injected with 15% dextrose had a significantly larger cross-sectional area compared with injured and noninjured saline-injected controls.[19] P2G solution has received the least research attention; although it is in active clinical use, no animal or in vitro study has assessed P2G effect using an injury model. Most clinicians report using these solutions as single agents, although concentration varies. In clinical practice, physicians sometimes mix prolotherapy solutions or use solutions serially in a single injection session depending on experience and local practice patterns. Neither effect of varied concentration nor mixtures have been assessed in basic science or clinical studies and no clinical trial has compared different solutions against one another.

CLINICAL EVIDENCE
Early Research

Since its inception, prolotherapy has been primarily used outside of academic centers. This has led to a pragmatic orientation of existing prolotherapy studies and a relative paucity of major rigorous clinical trials despite significant clinical activity. Although the first randomized controlled trial (RCT) did not appear until 1987, clinicians have enthusiastically reported the results of more modest, pilot-level clinical trials.

A 2005 systematic review of prolotherapy for all indications found 42 published reports of clinical prolotherapy trials since 1937.[20] Thirty-six of the studies were case reports and case series that included 3928 patients aged from 12 to 88 years. These uncontrolled studies provide the earliest and most clinically-oriented evidence for prolotherapy. Each study reported positive findings for patients with chronic, painful, refractory conditions. Report quality of the included studies varied widely; their internal methodological strength was generally consistent with publication date. The older case studies documented injectants and methods that are no longer in use. Contemporary solutions were noted to start with P2G in the 1960s, dextrose in the 1980s, and morrhuate sodium in the early 1990s. The case reports and case series highlighted that, over time, prolotherapy has been used and studied for a growing set of clinical indications. These case studies have also been used as pilot studies to develop new assessment techniques that could help elucidate the pathophysiology of a given condition[7] and test methodology for future, more robust randomized trials.[21] In general, although lacking control groups and randomization, these pragmatic studies[22] had the advantage of assessing effectiveness of prolotherapy in "real life settings" that patients encounter, including the prolotherapist's ability to select the patient and to individually tailor the injection protocol. Most subjects (72%, 2691 of 3741) assessed in the early literature were treated for LBP. However, other indications assessed by these early studies included knee OA, shoulder dislocation, neck strain, costochondritis, lateral epicondylosis (LE), and fibromyalgia.

Contemporary Research

Since the mid 1980s, research on prolotherapy effects has accelerated, with a dramatic increase in number and improvement in methodological quality of studies assessing prolotherapy (**Fig. 1**).

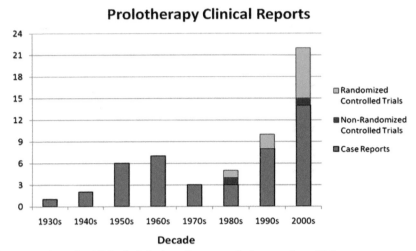

Fig. 1. Number of published clinical studies on prolotherapy since 1937.

To date, prolotherapy has been best assessed as a treatment for LBP, OA, and tendinopathy, each of which is a significant cause of pain and disability and is often refractory to best standard-of-care therapies. The severity and prevalence of each condition is age-related. Because the US population is aging, finding new effective therapies for these conditions can have an impact on individual patient care and overall public health. Prolotherapy has also been assessed as a treatment for nonspecific, nonsurgical LBP, OA of the knee and hand, and for several tendinopathies, including LE and Achilles, adductor, and plantar fasciitis. The following sections give a brief description of studies assessing prolotherapy for these clinical indications and level of evidence associated with each condition; this information is additionally summarized in **Table 1**.

LBP

LBP is among the most common reason patients see a primary care provider. Approximately 80% of Americans experience LBP during their lifetime. An estimated 15% to 20% of patients develop protracted pain, and approximately 2% to 8% experience chronic pain. LBP is second only to the common cold as a cause of lost work time. Productivity losses from chronic LBP approach $28 billion annually in the United States.[31]

Nonspecific LBP

Four RCTs evaluated prolotherapy for musculoskeletal LBP; 3 used P2G as the injectant[23,24,32] and the fourth used dextrose.[25] Each study used a protocol involving injections to the ligamentous insertions of the L4-S1 spinous processes, sacrum, and ilium. Although outcome measures varied, a common measure was the percentage of participants reporting more than 50% improvement in pain/disability scores at 6 months.

Two of these 4 RCTs reported positive findings compared with control injections. Ongley and colleagues[32] and Klein and colleagues[23] compared the treatment effects of prolotherapy combined with an adjunctive treatment with injected steroids, spinal manipulation, and exercise. In the Ongley study,[32] the intervention and control groups differed markedly on the makeup of initial injections and type of spinal manipulation

Table 1
Strength of evidence for prolotherapy as a treatment for chronic musculoskeletal conditions

Key Clinical Recommendation on Prolotherapy	Evidence Rating	References
Nonspecific LBP: may be effective; conflicting results in several RCTs	B	23–26
Sacroiliac joint dysfunction: may be effective in patients with documented failure of load transfer (disability) at the sacroiliac joint	B	27
Coccygodynia: may be effective based on prospective case series	B	28
LE: probably effective based on strong positive data in these small RCTs	A	6,7
Achilles tendinopathy: may be effective based on high quality prospective case series	B	9
Plantar fasciitis: may be effective, based on high-quality prospective case series	B	29
OA: may be effective for knee and finger OA, based on RCTs of moderately strong methodological quality	B	17,30

associated with the injections. Significantly more subjects in the prolotherapy (88%) group reported at least 50% reduction in pain severity compared with controls (39%). Also, prolotherapy subjects reported significantly decreased pain and disability levels compared with controls.[32] Klein and colleagues[23] used more similar treatment protocols in the 2 assessed groups, with subjects in both groups receiving steroid injections and spinal manipulation before prolotherapy. Again, significantly more prolotherapy subjects improved by 50% or more on pain or disability scores (77%) than controls (53%). Pain grid scores were also significantly lower in the prolotherapy group, with individual pain ($P = .06$) and disability ($P = .07$) scores trending toward significance compared with the control group.

Two of the 4 RCTs reported negative outcomes compared with control injections.[24,25] Dechow and colleagues[24] implemented a refined study protocol; subjects in both groups underwent 3 injection therapy sessions without adjacent spinal manipulation or physical therapy. Although both groups showed a trend toward improved severity scores on pain questionnaire, pain grid, and somatic perception measures, these changes did not reach statistical significance over time within or between groups. At 6 months, improvements in both groups were smaller than those of the other RCTs. Yelland and colleagues[25] have conducted the largest and most methodologically rigorous prolotherapy study published to date. Study subjects (N = 110), with an average of 14 years of LBP, were randomized to one of 4 intervention groups: dextrose and physical therapy, dextrose and "normal activity," saline injections ("control" injection) and physical therapy, or saline injections and normal activity. By 12 months, subjects in all groups reported improved pain (26%–44%) and disability (30%–44%) scores, without significant differences between groups. Most subjects (55%) stated that their improvement in pain and disability had been worth the effort of undergoing the intervention. The percentage of subjects who reached at least 50% pain reduction varied between 36% and 46% though these differences were not statistically significant.

Overall, interpretation of findings from these 4 RCTs is challenging. Both experimental and control groups received different treatment protocols, and none of the trials was designed to elicit a possible mechanism of prolotherapy action. Therefore, it is impossible to attribute effects to prolotherapy or any other specific intervention. A recent Cochrane Collaboration systematic review[26] did not find sufficient evidence to recommend prolotherapy for nonspecific LBP. However, these 4 RCTs present promising results overall, calling for well-designed, sufficiently powered research. All RCTs report improvements for pain and disability in all treatment groups consisting of subjects with chronic, moderate-to-severe LBP. In particular, Yelland and colleagues[25] reported clinical improvement in excess of minimal clinically important difference[33–35] and in excess of subjects' own perception of the minimum improvement necessary for prolotherapy to be worthwhile (25% for pain and 35% for disability).[21,25]

LBP due to specific causes

Prolotherapy research methods for LBP have been evolving amid much debate surrounding effectiveness, indications, treatment protocols, and solution types.[36,37] Given the promising aspects of the RCTs discussed earlier for nonspecific LBP combined with anecdotal clinical success, later clinical research has begun to assess prolotherapy in patients with more specific forms of LBP and loss of function in an effort to determine specific causes of LBP for which prolotherapy may be most effective.

Cusi and colleagues[27] assessed 25 subjects with sacroiliac joint dysfunction and pain refractory to 6 months or more of physical therapy and with documented failure of load transfer (disability) at the sacroiliac joint. They used a strong prolotherapy solution of 18% dextrose, delivered in 3 sets of injections over 12 weeks. Compared with baseline, pain and disability scores on 3 multidimensional outcome measures significantly improved at 26-month follow-up in excess of minimal clinically important difference.

Khan and colleagues[28] assessed 37 subjects with refractory coccygodynia. Using 25% dextrose in up to 3 prolotherapy injection sessions over 2 months, average pain scores, evaluated using a 0 to 10 visual analog scale (VAS), significantly decreased from a baseline score of 8.5 to 2.5 points at 2 months, far in excess of reported minimal clinically important difference for chronic pain.[38] The authors reported "good" pain relief for 30 of 37 subjects, and no improvement for the remaining 7.

In an especially novel study, Miller and colleagues[39] assessed prolotherapy for leg pain due to moderate-to-severe degenerative disc disease as determined by computed tomographic discography. Subjects (N = 76) who failed physical therapy and had substantial but temporary pain relief with 2 fluoroscopically guided epidural steroid injections were included. After an average of 3.5 sessions of biweekly, fluoroscopically-guided injections to the relevant disc space with 25% dextrose with bupivacaine, 43% of responders showed a significant, sustained treatment response of 71% improvement in pain score, with VAS score for responders at 8.9 (±1.4), 2.5 (±2.0), and 2.6 (±2.2) at baseline, 2, and 18 months, respectively. Although these 3 recent studies of prolotherapy for "specific" LBP were uncontrolled, they suggest the need for future RCTs with more focused clinical indications of axial pain and disability.

Tendinopathies

The strongest data supporting the efficacy of prolotherapy for any musculoskeletal condition compared with control injections are for chronic, painful tendon-overuse conditions that were formerly called tendonitis and are now more correctly termed tendinosis or tendinopathy to reflect existing, underlying pathophysiology.[40] Patients with tendinopathies commonly present to primary care providers and various medical specialists.[41,42] Tendinopathies are sometimes discussed as a group because the current understanding of overuse tendinopathies identifies them as sharing underlying noninflammatory pathology resulting from a repetitive motion or overuse injury and associated with painful degenerative tissue. Histopathology of tendon biopsies in patients undergoing surgery for painful tendinopathy reveals collagen separation[43]— thin, frayed, and fragile tendon fibrils, separated from each other lengthwise and disrupted in cross section and increase in tenocytes with myofibroblastic differentiation (tendon repair cells)—proteoglycan ground substance, and neovascularization. Classic inflammatory cells are usually absent.[43] Although this aspect of tendinosis was first described 25 years ago[44] and content experts have advocated a change in nomenclature (from tendonitis to tendinosis),[40] the use of the misnomer, tendonitis, continues.[45] Prolotherapy has been assessed as a treatment for 4 tendon disorders: LE, hip adductor, Achilles tendinopathy, and plantar fasciitis.

LE (tennis elbow) is an important common condition of the upper extremity with an incidence of 4 to 7per 1000 patients per year in primary care settings.[46–48] Its greatest impact is on workers with repetitive and high-load upper extremity tasks and on athletes. Its most common cause may be low-load, high-repetition activities, such as keyboarding, though formal data are lacking.[49] Cost and time away from job or activity are significant.[50,51] Although many nonsurgical therapies have been tested for LE refractory to conservative measures, none have demonstrated uniform effectiveness in the long term.[52–54] Scarpone and colleagues[8] conducted an RCT to determine whether prolotherapy improves self-reported elbow pain, and objectively measured grip strength and extension strength in patients with chronic LE. Twenty adults with at least 6 months of moderately-to-severely painful LE refractory to rest, nonsteroidal anti-inflammatory medications (NSAIDs), and corticosteroid injections, were randomized to prolotherapy with dextrose and morrhuate sodium (1 part 5% sodium morrhuate, 1.5 parts 50% dextrose, 0.5 parts 4% lidocaine, 0.5 parts 0.5% bupivacaine hydrochloride (Sensorcaine), and 3.5 parts normal saline) or control injections with normal saline. Three prolotherapy sessions were administered, with injection at the supracondylar ridge, lateral epicondyle, and annular ligament. Compared with controls, prolotherapy subjects reported significantly decreased pain scores at 8 and 16 weeks. These pain score differences between the groups were associated with a significant improvement in prolotherapy subjects (from 5.1 ± 0.8 at baseline, down to 0.5 ± 0.4 at 16 weeks), whereas the controls did not report significant change (4.5 ± 1.7 to 3.5 ± 1.5). In addition to pain reduction, prolotherapy subjects also showed significantly improved isometric strength compared with controls and grip strength compared with baseline. These clinical improvements seen in prolotherapy subjects were maintained at 52 weeks.

Achilles tendinopathy is a common overuse injury seen in athletes and in the general population. This painful condition is a cause of considerable distress and disability.[55] Maxwell and colleagues[7] conducted a well-designed case series to assess whether prolotherapy, administered during a mean of 4 injection sessions, at 6-week intervals, would decrease pain in 36 adults with painful Achilles tendinopathy. In this study, 25% dextrose solution was injected into hypoechoic regions of the Achilles tendon under ultrasonographic guidance. In addition to self-reported measures, the investigators also assessed ultrasonography-based tendon thickness and the degree of hypoechogenicity and neovascularity—ultrasonographic findings recently reported to correlate to tendinopathy severity.[56,57] At 52 weeks, prolotherapy-treated subjects reported decrease in VAS-assessed pain severity by 88%, 84%, and 78% during rest, "usual activity", and sport, respectively. In addition, tendon thickness decreased significantly. The overall grade of tendon pathology, hypoechoic and anechoic tendon regions, and neovascularity were all improved in some, but not all, subjects who reported clinical improvement. Therefore, the relationship between ultrasonographically assessed characteristics and the degree of clinical improvement remains unclear.

Hip adductor tendinopathy associated with groin pain is a common problem among those who engage in kicking sports.[58] Topol and colleagues[59] conducted a case series assessing prolotherapy for chronic groin pain, a condition involving pain and tenderness at tendon and ligament insertions in the groin area. Male athletes (N = 24), with an average duration of 15.5 months of groin pain despite standard therapy were injected with 12.5% dextrose at the thigh and suprapubic abdominal insertions of the adductor tendon and at the symphysis pubis at 4-week intervals until pain resolved or subjects had no improvement for 2 consecutive sessions. On average, subjects received 3 prolotherapy sessions. At a mean of 17 months, subjects reported dramatic significant improvements on 2 pain scales (VAS and the Nirschl pain phase scale). Of 24 subjects, 20 had no pain and 22 returned to sports without restrictions after therapy.

Plantar fasciitis is a common injury among athletes engaged in sports requiring running and among general primary-care patients. It is reported to account for 15% of all adult foot complaints requiring professional consultation, and in a 2002 survey of running-related injuries, plantar fasciitis was the third most prevalent injury.[60,61] Among standard-of-care approaches, there is limited evidence for the effectiveness of any one treatment for plantar fasciitis, including steroid injections.[29] Ryan and colleagues[30] assessed prolotherapy for chronic plantar fasciitis refractory to conservative care. Twenty adults with an average of 21 months of heal pain underwent ultrasound-guided 25% dextrose injections for an average of 3 treatment sessions delivered at 6-week intervals. Pain scores were assessed using a 100-point VAS at baseline and at 11.8 months. Pain severity significantly improved at rest, during activities of daily living, and during sporting activities by 26.5, 49.7, and 56.5 points, respectively compared with baseline, and 16 of 20 subjects reported good or excellent treatment effects.

OA

Prolotherapy has been assessed as a treatment for knee and finger OA[16,62] and is the subject of ongoing studies.[63] Arthritis is a leading cause of disability in the world and in the United States where it affects 43 million persons.[64–66] OA is the most common form of arthritis and the most common joint disorder.[67] In the United States, symptomatic knee OA is present in up to 6% of the population older than 30 years,[67] and it has an overall incidence of 360,000 cases per year.[68] Incidence increases up to 10-fold from ages 30 to 65 years and more thereafter.[69] OA results in a high burden of disease and substantial economic impact through its high prevalence, time lost off work, and frequent use of health care resources.[64,70]

Allopathic and CAM treatment recommendations for OA have been published, aimed at modifiable risk factor correction, symptom control, and disease modification.[71,72] Although these modalities may help some patients, none has been proven to provide definitive pain control or disease modification for patients with knee OA. The Agency for Research Health and Quality has recently evaluated the most common standard treatment options, including glucosamine, chondroitin, viscosupplementation, and arthroscopic debridement.[73] These have not demonstrated effectiveness compared with placebo. The high burden of knee OA and the absence of a cure continue to stimulate intense search for new agents to modify disease and control symptoms.

Reeves and colleagues[16,62] assessed prolotherapy as a treatment for knee and finger OA. Subjects with finger or knee pain and radiological evidence of OA were randomly assigned to receive 3 injection sessions of prolotherapy with 10% dextrose and lidocaine or lidocaine and bacteriostatic water (control group). In the finger OA trial, intervention subjects significantly improved in "pain-with-movement" and "flexion-range" scores compared with controls; pain scores at rest and with grip showed a tendency to improvement, without reaching statistical significance. In the knee OA trial, subjects in both groups reported significant improvements in pain and swelling scores, number of buckling episodes, and flexion range of motion compared with baseline, but without statistically significant differences between the groups. Twelve-month follow-up in both studies included improved radiological features of OA on plain radiographic films: investigators reported decreased joint space narrowing and osteophytic grade in the finger study and increased patellofemoral cartilage thickness in the knee study. These radiological findings may suggest disease modification properties of prolotherapy. Whether or not subjects in the knee study had a baseline concomitant meniscal pathology was not reported or included in entry criteria. Furthermore, the ability of plain radiograph to quantify patellofemoral cartilage thickness is questionable, limiting impact of these findings.

CONTRAINDICATIONS, SIDE EFFECTS AND ADVERSE EVENTS
Contraindications

Absolute contraindications to prolotherapy are few and include acute infections such as cellulitis, local abscess, or septic arthritis. Relative contraindications include acute gouty arthritis and acute fracture.

Common Side Effects

The main risk of prolotherapy is pain and mild bleeding caused by needle trauma. At the time of injections, patients frequently report pain, a sense of fullness, and occasional numbness at the injection site. These side effects are typically self-limited. A postinjection pain flare during the first 72 hours after the injections is common clinically, but its incidence has not been well documented. An ongoing study of prolotherapy for knee OA pain has noted that 10% to 20% of subjects experience such flares.[74] Pain flares are likewise typically self-limited, and usually respond well to acetaminophen (500–650 mg every 4 hours as needed). On rare occasions, the occurrence of strong, postinjection pain may require treatment with narcotic medication. NSAIDs are not routinely used after the procedure but may be indicated if the pain does not resolve with other measures. Most patients with pain flares experience diminution of pain in 5 to 7 days after injections; regular activities can be resumed at this time.

Adverse Events

Although prolotherapy performed by an experienced injector seems safe, the injection of ligaments, tendons, and joints with irritant solutions raises safety concerns. Theoretical risks of prolotherapy injections include lightheadedness, allergic reaction, and infection or neurologic (nerve) damage. Injections should be performed using universal precautions and the patient should be prone if possible. Dextrose is extremely safe; it is Food and Drug Administration (FDA)-approved for intravenous treatment of hypoglycemia and for caloric supplementation. Morrhuate sodium is a vascular sclerosant used in gastrointestinal procedures and vein sclerosing. Allergic reactions to morrhuate sodium are rare. Although P2G is not FDA-approved for any indication, it has not been reported in clinical trials to cause significant side effects or adverse events.

Historically, a small number of significant, prolotherapy-related complications have been reported. They were associated with perispinal injections for back or neck pain using very concentrated solutions, and they included 5 cases of neurologic impairment from spinal cord irritation[75–77] and 1 death in 1959 following prolotherapy with zinc sulfate for LBP.[75] Neither zinc sulfate nor concentrated prolotherapy solutions are currently in general use. In a survey of 95 clinicians using prolotherapy, there were 29 reports of pneumothoraces after prolotherapy for back and neck pain, two of which required hospitalization for a chest tube, and 14 cases of allergic reactions, although none classified as serious.[5] A later survey of practicing prolotherapists yielded similar results for spinal prolotherapy: spinal headache, pneumothoraces, nerve damage, and nonsevere spinal cord insult and disc injury were reported.[78] The investigators concluded that these events were no more common in prolotherapy than for other spinal injection procedures. No serious side effects or adverse events were reported for prolotherapy when used for peripheral joint indications.

PRACTICAL PROLOTHERAPY
Incorporating Prolotherapy into Practice

Similar to corticosteroid injections, prolotherapy is an unregulated procedure without certification by any governing body. Formal training is not provided by most medical schools, residencies, and fellowships. However, to be performed appropriately and safely, prolotherapy requires specialized training. In the United States, it is taught to physicians and other health-care providers (authorized to deliver joint-type injections) in semiformal workshops and formal CME by several organizations, including university settings (**Table 2**).

Patients and physicians who desire consultation for prolotherapy may have difficulty finding an appropriate consulting prolotherapist. Online resources (see **Table 2**) are available that can help locate a prolotherapist, although information is limited by lack of a credentialing structure and governing body for prolotherapy.

Despite limited institutional support, interest in prolotherapy is increasing, and it is performed in increasing numbers, primarily in 2 settings. For several decades, prolotherapy has been mostly performed outside of mainstream medicine by independent physicians. Later, multispecialty groups that include family or sports medicine physicians, physiatrists, orthopedic surgeons, neurologists, or anesthesiologists have been incorporating prolotherapy because of positive clinical experience and research reports. Prolotherapy is one of several injection therapies that may promote healing of chronically injured soft tissue. Other therapies receiving active clinical and research attention for chronic musculoskeletal pain include whole blood, platelet rich plasma, and polidocanol injections.[9] In both settings, prolotherapy is viewed as a valued procedure, primarily reserved for patients who have failed other treatments or those who are not surgical candidates.

The Authors' Clinic

The authors practice in a community in which several primary care physicians and specialists perform prolotherapy; receptivity to prolotherapy in the authors' setting is growing. Some health insurance plans in the author's area cover prolotherapy for

Table 2
Educational and informational prolotherapy resources

Name/URL	Comments
The Anatomy, Diagnosis, and Treatment of Chronic Myofascial Pain with Prolotherapy http://www.ocpd.wisc.edu/Course_Catalog/	CME on the basics of prolotherapy. This 3.5 d conference is offered through the University of Wisconsin School of Medicine and Public Health. All aspects of clinical and research aspects of prolotherapy are covered.
Hackett-Hemwall Foundation list of prolotherapists http://www.hacketthemwall.org/HHF/List_of_Prolotherapists.html	The Hackett-Hemwall Foundation is a nonprofit medical foundation whose mission is to provide high-quality treatment of musculoskeletal problems to underserved people around the world. Physicians listed on the site have completed the foundation's high-volume CME experience in prolotherapy.
Commercial prolotherapy physician listing http://www.getprolo.com	This site lists physicians by state who perform prolotherapy. It includes contact information, a short biography, and prolotherapy credentials. Physicians pay to list themselves on this site.
AAOM http://www.aaomed.org	The AAOM is a nonprofit organization that provides information and educational programs on comprehensive nonsurgical musculoskeletal treatment, including prolotherapy. This searchable site lists AAOM members who perform prolotherapy.

Abbreviation: AAOM, American Association of Orthopaedic Medicine.

the indications discussed. Referrals can be made similar to those for more conventional procedures. An initial consultation, including a complete history and physical, is performed by the prolotherapist to determine if the patient is a candidate for prolotherapy. If so, side effects, adverse events, and expected course of injections are explained, and the patient is asked to sign a procedure consent form. Information is also provided to patients in written form. (**Table 3**) The patient is then scheduled for up to 3 outpatient prolotherapy sessions, typically 4 to 6 weeks apart. At each subsequent visit, an interval history is obtained and physical examination is performed. If the patient does not report improvement after 3 prolotherapy sessions, alternative interventions are pursued.

CLINICAL RECOMMENDATIONS

Present data suggest that prolotherapy is probably an effective therapy for painful overuse tendinopathy. Specifically, Scarpone and colleagues[8] provide level A evidence for prolotherapy as an effective therapy for LE. Subjects with refractory LE and treated with prolotherapy reported significant reduction in pain and improved isometric strength compared with those who received control injections. These findings are supported by the Maxwell,[7] Topol[59] and Ryan[30] studies that report strong case series results for Achilles, hip adductor, and plantar fasciitis, respectively and provide level B evidence for these conditions. Given that the underlying mechanism

Table 3 Prolotherapy at a glance	
Definition of prolotherapy	Prolotherapy is an injection-based CAM therapy for chronic musculoskeletal pain. This treatment aims to stimulate a natural healing response at the site of painful soft tissue and joints.
What is involved	Prolotherapy treatment typically involves getting a series of 2–5 monthly injections of a topical anesthetic and a solution of other medicines directly on sore tendon or ligaments or into painful joints.
Conditions for which it is used and is it effective	Prolotherapy is generally used for musculoskeletal pain of more than 3 mo. Conditions that have responded well to prolotherapy in published studies include tennis elbow, Achilles tendinopathy, and other overuse injuries involving tendons. Prolotherapy is also probably effective for knee OA and LBP, although studies assessing these conditions are less conclusive.
Safety	Studies indicate that prolotherapy is safe when performed by an experienced practitioner. It does not seem to have a greater risk than other injection techniques, such as steroid injections.
Pain	No one loves getting a shot, although prolotherapy injections typically hurt less than most immunizations. Most patients tolerate prolotherapy injection-related pain well with only topical and conservative measures. Physicians can pretreat with a pain reliever if necessary.

of injury and pathophysiologic effects are similar for tendinopathies, prolotherapy is also a reasonable option for these conditions. Randomized controlled trials for all 3 and other tendinopathies are indicated.

Recommendations are more difficult to make for OA and LBP, both of which are associated with more complex anatomy and less clear pathophysiology than that seen in tendinopathies. Side effects and potential adverse events of prolotherapy are likely to be more serious when performed for spinal or intra-articular indications and must be weighed against the potential for improvement. Existing studies provide level B evidence that prolotherapy is effective for nonspecific LBP compared with a patient's baseline condition. Given that subjects with refractory, disabling LBP significantly improved compared with their own baseline status in the Yelland study,[25] patients may reasonably try prolotherapy when performed by an experienced injector. Future studies with more focused inclusion criteria may help determine which specific low back pathologies respond to prolotherapy. Existing studies provide level B evidence that prolotherapy is effective for knee and finger OA compared with control injections.[16,62] Prolotherapy by an experienced physician is a treatment modality worth considering by primary care physicians for these conditions, especially when they are refractory to more conventional therapy.

ACKNOWLEDGMENTS

Jeffrey Patterson, DO.

REFERENCES

1. Hackett GS, Hemwall GA, Montgomery GA. Ligament and tendon relaxation treated by prolotherapy. 5th edition. Oak Park (IL): Gustav A. Hemwall; 1993.
2. Linetsky FS, FRafael M, Saberski L. Pain management with regenerative injection therapy (RIT). In: Weiner RS, editor. Pain management. Boca Raton (FL): CRC Press; 2002. p. 381–402.
3. Matthews JH. Nonsurgical treatment of pain in lumbar spinal stenosis. [letter to the editor]. Am Fam Physician 1999;59(2):280–4.
4. Schnirring L. Are your patients asking about prolotherapy? Physician Sports Med 2000;28(8):15–7.
5. Dorman TA. Prolotherapy: a survey. J Orthopaedic Med 1993;15(2):49–50.
6. Linetsky FS, Botwin K, Gorfin L, et al. Regeneration injection therapy (RIT): effectiveness and appropriate usage. Florida Academy of Pain Medicine; 2001. Available at: http://www.gracermedicalgroup.com/resources/articles/rf_file_0025.pdf. Accessed October 15, 2009.
7. Maxwell NJ, Ryan MB, Taunton JE, et al. Sonographically guided intratendinous injection of hyperosmolar dextrose to treat chronic tendinosis of the Achilles tendon: a pilot study. Am J Roentgenol 2007;189(4):W215–20.
8. Scarpone M, Rabago D, Zgierska A, et al. The efficacy of prolotherapy for lateral epicondylosis: a pilot study. Clin J Sport Med 2008;18:248–54.
9. Rabago D, Best TM, Zgierska A, et al. A systematic review of four injection therapies for lateral epicondylosis: prolotherapy, polidocanol, whole blood and platelet rich plasma. Br J Sports Med 2009. DOI:10.1136/bjsm.2008.052761.
10. Liu YK, Tipton CM, Matthes RD, et al. An in-situ study of the influence of a sclerosing solution in rabbit medial collateral ligaments and its junction strength. Connect Tissue Res 1983;11:95–102.
11. Maynard JA, Pedrini VA, Pedrini-Mille A, et al. Morphological and biochemical effects of sodium morrhuate on tendons. J Orthop Res 1985;3:236–48.
12. Banks A. A rationale for prolotherapy. J Orthop Med 1991;13(3):54–9.
13. Hoksrud A, Ohberg L, Alfredson H, et al. Ultrasound-guided sclerosis of neovessels in painful chronic patellar tendinopathy. Am J Sports Med 2006;34:1738–46.
14. Zeisig E, Fahlström M, Ohberg L, et al. A 2-year sonographic follow-up after intratendinous injection therapy in patients with tennis elbow. Br J Sports Med 2008. DOI:10.1136/bjsm.2008.049874.
15. Kim SR, Stitik TP, Foye PM. Critical review of prolotherapy for osteoarthritis, low back pain, and other musculoskeletal conditions: a physiatric perspective. Am J Phys Med Rehabil 2004;83(5):379–89.
16. Reeves KD, Hassanein K. Randomized prospective double-blind placebo-controlled study of dextrose prolotherapy for knee osteoarthritis with or without ACL laxity. Altern Ther Health Med 2000;6(2):68–80.
17. Jensen K, Rabago D, Best TM, et al. Early inflammatory response of knee ligaments to prolotherapy in a rat model. J Orthop Res 2008;26:816–23.
18. Aneja A, Spero G, Weinhold P, et al. Suture plication, thermal shrinkage and sclerosing agents. Am J Sports Med 2005;33:1729–34.
19. Jensen KT. Healing response of knee ligaments to prolotherapy in a rat model [PhD dissertation]. Madison (WI): Biomedical Engineering, University of Wisconsin; 2006.

20. Rabago D, Best T, Beamsly M, et al. A systematic review of prolotherapy for chronic musculoskeletal pain. Clin J Sport Med 2005;15(5):376–80.

21. Yelland M, Yeo M, Schluter P. Prolotherapy injections for chronic low back pain: results of a pilot comparative study. Australian Musculoskeletal Medicine 2000; 5(2):20–30. Available at: http://www.musmed.com/.

22. Ernst E, Pittler MH, Stevinson C, et al. Randomised clinical trials: pragmatic or fastidious? Focus on Alternative and Complementary Therapies 2001;63(3):179–80. Available at: http://www.pharmpress.com/shop/journals.asp?a=1&cid=27.

23. Klein RG, Eek BC, DeLong WB, et al. A randomized double-blind trial of dextrose-glycerine-phenol injections for chronic, low back pain. J Spinal Disord 1993;6(1): 23–33.

24. Dechow E, Davies RK, Carr AJ, et al. A randomized, double-blind, placebo-controlled trial of sclerosing injections in patients with chronic low back pain. Rheumatology 1999;38:1255–9.

25. Yelland M, Glasziou P, Bogduk N, et al. Prolotherapy injections, saline injections, and exercises for chronic low back pain: a randomized trial. Spine 2004;29(1):9–16.

26. Yelland MJ, Del Mar C, Pirozo S, et al. Prolotherapy injections for chronic low back pain: a systematic review. Spine 2004;29:2126–33.

27. Cusi M, Saunders J, Hungerford B, et al. The use of prolotherapy in the sacro-iliac joint. Br J Sports Med 2008. DOI:10.1136/bjsm.2007.042044.

28. Khan SA, Kumar A, Varshney MK, et al. Dextrose prolotherapy for recalcitrant coccygodynia. J Orthop Surg 2008;16:27–9.

29. Crawford F, Thomson C. Interventions for treating plantar heel pain. Cochrane Database Syst Rev 2003;(3):CD000416.

30. Ryan MB, Wong AD, Gillies JH, et al. Sonographically guided intratendinous injections of hyperosmolar dextrose/lidocaine: a pilot study for the treatment of chronic plantar fasciitis. Br J Sports Med 2009;43:303–6. DOI: 10.1136/bjsm.2008.050021.

31. Wheeler AH. Pathophysiology of chronic back pain. Available at: http://www.emedicine.com/neuro/topic516.htm; 2007.

32. Ongley MJ, Klein RG, Dorman TA, et al. A new approach to the treatment of chronic low back pain. Lancet 1987;2:143–6.

33. Bellamy N, Carr A, Dougados M, et al. Towards a definition of "difference" in osteoarthritis. J Rheumatol 2001;28(2):427–30.

34. Redelmeier DA, Guyatt GH, Goldstein RS. Assessing the minimal important difference in symptoms: a comparison of two techniques. J Clin Epidemiol 1996;49: 1215–9.

35. Wells GA, Tugwell P, Kraag GR, et al. Minimum important difference between patients with rheumatoid arthritis: the patient's perspective. J Rheumatol 1993; 20:557–60.

36. Loeser JD. Point of view. Spine 2004;29(1):16.

37. Reeves KD, Klein RG, DeLong WB. Letter to the editor. Spine 2004;29(16): 1839–40.

38. Farrar JT, Young JP, LaMoreaux L, et al. Clinical importance of changes in chronic pain intensity measured on an 11-point numerical rating scale. Pain 2001;94: 149–58.

39. Miller MR, Mathews RS, Reeves KD. Treatment of painful advanced internal lumbar disc derangement with intradiscal injection of hypertonic dextrose. Pain Physician 2006;9:115–21.

40. Khan KM, Cook JL, Kannus P, et al. Time to abandon the 'tendinitis' myth. BMJ 2002;324:626–7.

41. Bongers PM. The cost of shoulder pain at work. Variation in work tasks and good job opportunities are essential for prevention. BMJ 2001;322:64–5.
42. Wilson JJ, Best TM. Common overuse tendon problems: a review and recommendations for treatment. Am Fam Physician 2005;72:811–8.
43. Khan KM, Cook JL, Bonar F, et al. Histopathology of tendinopathies. Update and implications for clinical management. Sports Med 1999;27:393–408.
44. Puddu G, Ippolito E, Postacchini FA. classification of Achilles tendon disease. Am J Sports Med 1976;4:145–50.
45. Johnson GW, Cadwallader K, Scheffel SB, et al. Treatment of lateral epicondylitis. Am Fam Physician 2007;76:843–8, 849–50; 853.
46. Verhar J. Tennis elbow: anatomical, epidemiological and therapeutic aspects. Int Orthop 1994;18:263–7.
47. Hamilton P. The prevalence of humeral epicondylitis: a survey in general practice. J R Coll Gen Pract 1986;36:464–5.
48. Kivi P. The etiology and conservative treatment of lateral epicondylitis. Scand J Rehabil Med 1983;15:37–41.
49. Gabel GT. Acute and chronic tendinopathies at the elbow. Curr Opin Rheumatol 1999;11:138–48.
50. Ono Y, Nakamura R, Shimaoka M, et al. Epicondylitis among cooks in nursery schools. Occup Environ Med 1998;55:172–9.
51. Ritz BR. Humeral epicondylitis among gas and waterworks employees. Scand J Work Environ Health 1995;21:478–86.
52. Buchbinder R, Green S, White M, et al. Shock wave therapy for lateral elbow pain. Cochrane Database Syst Rev 2002;1:CD003524.
53. Smidt N, van der Windt DA, Assendelft WJ, et al. Corticosteroid injections, physiotherapy, or a wait-and-see policy for lateral epicondylitis: a randomised controlled trial. Lancet 2002;359:657–62.
54. Struijs PA, Smidt N, Arola H, et al. Orthotic devices for the treatment of tennis elbow. Cochrane Database Syst Rev 2005;(3).
55. Kvist M. Achilles tendon injuries in athletes. Sports Med 1994;18:173–201.
56. Zeisig E, Ohberg L, Alfredson H. Extensor origin vascularity related to pain in patients with tennis elbow. Knee Surg Sports Traumatol Arthrosc 2006;14:659–63.
57. Alfredson H, Ohberg L. Sclerosing injections to areas of neovascularization reduce pain in chronic Achilles tendinopathy: a double-blind randomised trial. Knee Surg Sports Traumatol Arthrosc 2005;13:338–44.
58. Holmich P, Uhrskou P, Ulnits L. Effectiveness of active physical training as treatment of long-standing adductor-related groin pain in athletes: a randomized controlled trial. Lancet 1999;353:439–43.
59. Topol GA, Reeves KD, Hassanein KM. Efficacy of dextrose prolotherapy in elite male kicking-sport athletes with groin pain. Arch Phys Med Rehabil 2005;86:697–702.
60. Buchbinder R. Plantar fasciitis. N Engl J Med 2004;350:2159–66.
61. Taunton J, Ryan M, Clement D, et al. A retrospective case-control analysis of 2002 running injuries. Br J Sports Med 2002;36:95–101.
62. Reeves KD, Hassanein K. Randomized, prospective, placebo-controlled double-blind study of dextrose prolotherapy for osteoarthritic thumb and finger (DIP, PIP, and Trapeziometacarpal) joints: evidence of clinical efficacy. J Altern Complement Med 2000;6(4):311–20.
63. Rabago D. The efficacy of prolotherapy in osteoarthritic knee pain. NIH-NCCAM Grant, 1K23 AT001879–01; in press.

64. Reginster JY. The prevalence and burden of arthritis. Rheumatology 2002; 41(Suppl 1):3–6.
65. CDC. Prevalence and impact of chronic joint symptoms-seven states, 1996. MMWR Morb Mortal Wkly Rep 1998;47:345–51.
66. CDC. Prevalence of disabilities and associated health conditions-United States, 1991–1992. MMWR Morb Mortal Wkly Rep 1994;43:730–9.
67. Felson DT, Zhang Y. An update on the epidemiology of knee and hip osteoarthritis with a view to prevention. Arthritis Rheum 1998;41(8):1343–55.
68. Wilson MG, Michet CJ, Ilstrup DM, et al. Ideopathic symptomatic osteoarthritis of the hip and knee: a population-based incidence study. Mayo Clin Proc 1990;65: 1214–21.
69. Oliveria SA, Felson DT, Klein RA, et al. Estrogen replacement therapy and the development of osteoarthritis. Epidemiology 1996;7:415–9.
70. Levy E, Ferme A, Perocheau D, et al. [Socioeconomic costs of osteoarthritis in France]. Rev Rhum Ed Fr 1993;60:63S–7S [in French].
71. Felson DT, Lawarence RC, Hochberg MC, et al. Osteoarthritis: new insights, part 2: treatment approaches. Ann Intern Med 2000;133:726–37.
72. American College of Rheumatology Subcommittee on Osteoarthritis Guidelines. Recommendations for the medical management of osteoarthritis of the hip and knee. Arthritis Rheum 2000;43:1905–15.
73. Samson DJ, Grant MD, Ratko TA, et al. Treatment of primary and secondary osteoarthritis of the knee. Evid Rep Technol Assess (Full Rep) 2007;151. Available at: http://www.ncbi.hlm.nih.gov/pubmed/18088162. Accessed October 16, 2009.
74. Rabago D, Zgierska A, Mundt M, et al. Efficacy of prolotherapy for knee osteoarthritis: results of a prospective case series. Poster presentation at: North American Research Conference on Complementary and Integrative Medicine. May 9, 2009.
75. Schneider RC, Williams JJ, Liss L. Fatality after injection of sclerosing agent to precipitate fibro-osseous proliferation. JAMA 1959;170(15):1768–72.
76. Keplinger JE, Bucy PC. Paraplegia from treatment with sclerosing agents - report of a case. JAMA 1960;173(12):1333–6.
77. Hunt WE, Baird WC. Complications following injection of sclerosing agent to precipitate fibro-osseous proliferation. J Neurosurg 1961;18:461–5.
78. Dagenais S, Ogunseitan O, Haldeman S, et al. Side effects and adverse events related to intraligamentous injection of sclerosing solutions (prolotherapy) for back and neck pain: a survey of practitioners. Arch Phys Med Rehabil 2006; 87:909–13.

Meditation in Medical Practice: A Review of the Evidence and Practice

Luke Fortney, MD[a,b,*], Molly Taylor, BS[c]

KEYWORDS

- Meditation • Mindfulness • Stress • Burnout • Mind-body
- Medical education • Contemplation • Contemplative prayer

WHAT IS MEDITATION?

Found in cultures, spiritual traditions, and healing systems throughout the world, meditation is a mind-body practice with many methods and variations, all of which are grounded in the silence and stillness of compassionate, nonjudgmental present-moment awareness. Although contemplative meditation practices are largely rooted in the world's spiritual traditions, the practice of meditation does not require belief in any particular religious or cultural system. The increased research and familiarization of mindfulness meditation within the fields of neuroscience, psychology, and medicine have led to an increased understanding of consciousness and improved treatment for many health conditions.

Mindfulness is one aspect of the meditation experience that reflects the basic and fundamental human capacity to attend to relevant aspects of experience in a nonjudgmental and nonreactive way, which in turn cultivates clear thinking, equanimity, compassion, and openheartedness. According to University of Massachusetts Center for Mindfulness founder Jon Kabat-Zinn, "Meditation is simplicity itself. It's about stopping and being present. That is all." The stated goal of mindfulness is to maintain fluid awareness in a moment by moment experiential process that helps one disengage from strong attachment to beliefs, thoughts, or emotions in a way that generates greater sense of emotional balance and well-being.[1] This simple yet radical assertion holds the potential for wide-reaching therapeutic benefit for many current health care challenges such as rising health care costs,[2] chronic lifestyle-influenced illness,[3]

---

[a] Department of Family Medicine, University of Wisconsin-Madison, Madison, WI, USA
[b] UW Health Odana-Atrium Family Medicine Clinic, 5618 Odana Road, Madison, WI 53719, USA
[c] Dartmouth Medical School, USA
* Corresponding author. UW Health Odana-Atrium Family Medicine Clinic, 5618 Odana Road, Madison, WI 53719.
E-mail address: Luke.Fortney@fammed.wisc.edu (L. Fortney).

Prim Care Clin Office Pract 37 (2010) 81–90
doi:10.1016/j.pop.2009.09.004
0095-4543/10/$ – see front matter. Published by Elsevier Inc.

primarycare.theclinics.com

practitioner burnout,[4] patient dissatisfaction,[5] and generalized stress for the practitioner[6] and the patient.[7]

WHY MEDITATE?

Prescribed meditation practice can elicit physical ease and mental stability, which provide a foundation for health and wellness as they directly influence one's ability to meet the challenges resulting from stress, burnout, and illness for patient and practitioner alike. For most people, illness brings out feelings of confusion, anxiety, fear, and anger. Shock, isolation, depression, fear, and helplessness are some common experiences patients face when dealing with chronic disease.[8] Feeling out of control or losing one's ground can give rise to reactivity of the mind and body that leads to increased pain and suffering. Applying the simple practice of nonjudgmental present-moment awareness and experiencing how this process influences one's relationship with life stressors is one way that meditation practice addresses the epidemic of mind-body afflictions that are expressed physically, such as acid reflux, migraine headache, low back pain, restless legs, fibromyalgia, chronic fatigue, irritable bowel, and many other conditions. These and other conditions disproportionately burden health care systems and often do not respond to conventional treatment alone.[2] Mediation is an inward-orienting, self-empowering practice that can stimulate the healing process and help patients and health care practitioners navigate through unsettling and turbulent experiences. According to experienced meditation teacher Charlotte Joko Beck,[9] "The practice of meditation provides a skill that affords a greater sense of self-determination—the ability to cultivate and draw upon inner resources to help meet all circumstances with equanimity and clarity."

REVIEW OF MEDITATION RESEARCH

Evidence pointing to the medical benefits of meditation has been widely documented, and continues to increase in quality and quantity. In 2007 there were more than 70 scientific articles published on mindfulness meditation practice. In particular, the biologic correlates of meditation experience have received the most attention in research, quite out of proportion to the complete meditative experience, which includes objective external effects and subjective internal experience. However, research is only beginning to elucidate how the mind-body connection affects health in promoting wellness and managing and preventing disease.

The interplay between the mind and body has been difficult to describe and operationalize from a scientific standpoint. However, many examples reveal the potential value in developing clinically oriented mind-body therapies. As early as 1935, French cardiologist Brosse studied Indian yogis capable of decreasing their heart rates to almost 0 on electrocardiographic (ECG) recordings.[10] In 1961, Bagchi and Wenger[11] found that some meditation experts could produce bidirectional changes in every measurable autonomic variable. The Lancet published an account of the voluntary live burial of a yogi who sat cross-legged underground for 62 hours while continuous vital sign recordings revealed no distress.[12] Hoenig witnessed an experiment in 1968 where a yogi confined for 9 hours in a small enclosed pit and monitored with electroencephalography and an ECG showed a normal waking rhythm for the full 9 hours, leading the researchers to conclude that the subject was awake and relaxed throughout the experiment. They also observed a variable heart rate from 40 to 100 beats a minute in recurring cycles on ECG.[13] As in fetal heart monitoring, later research showed that synchronous increases in heart rate variability in adults predicts a decrease in cardiovascular mortality,[14,15] which can be reproduced using meditation practices.[16,17]

Benson helped pioneer an academic interest in meditation through his research on the physiologic and neurochemical principles of the relaxation response, which is defined as a hypometabolic state of parasympathetic activation.[18] Many studies have shown that meditation training reduces anxiety and increases positive affect,[19–21] whereas others show that mindfulness meditation prevents recurrence of depression.[22,23] In a 1985 study by Kabat-Zinn and colleagues,[24] patients with chronic pain showed a statistically significant reduction in various measures of pain symptoms when trained in MBSR. Meditation practices have shown beneficial effects in the treatment of tension headaches,[25] psoriasis,[26] blood pressure,[27–29] serum cholesterol,[29] smoking cessation,[30,31] alcohol abuse,[32] carotid atherosclerosis,[33] coronary artery disease,[3,34,35] longevity and cognitive function in the elderly,[36] psychiatric disorders,[18–23,37] excessive worry,[38] use of medical care,[39] and medical costs in treating chronic pain.[40] A 2004 meta-analysis found MBSR training useful for a broad range of difficult-to-treat chronic disorders such as depression, anxiety, fibromyalgia, mixed cancer diagnoses, coronary artery disease, chronic pain, obesity, and eating disorders. The authors noted consistent and strong effect sizes across these very different situations, indicating a generalized application of meditation for daily life distress and extraordinary medical disorders and Iverson.[41]

In a meta-analysis of brain imaging studies on various meditation styles, Newberg and Iversen[42] suggests that the neurophysiologic effects derived from various meditation practices seem to outline a consistent and reproducible pattern of significant brain activity in key cerebral structures. Research focusing more specifically on these physiologic effects of meditation by Davidson and colleagues[43] described a positive correlation between meditation practice and left-sided prefrontal cortex activity, which is associated with positive affect. In this study, mindfulness meditation was associated with increases in antibody titers to influenza vaccine suggesting correlation among meditation, positive emotional states, localized brain activity, and improved immune function. Corroborating research shows a direct link between immune function and mood, with positive affective states resulting in stronger immune function and decreased incidence of illness.[44–46] Lutz observed increased left-sided prefrontal cortex gamma wave activity and synchronicity in expert Tibetan Buddhist meditators with more than 10,000 hours of meditation experience compared with novice meditator controls, at rest and during meditation.[47] This finding suggests that attention and affective processes are flexible skills that can be learned.

Although ongoing research aims to elucidate the measurable biologic correlates of meditation and its significance to health, it is important to acknowledge the experiential knowledge that has arisen from time-tested practices of the great spiritual traditions. Meditation practitioners within these spiritual systems continue to explore the subtle inner dimensions of meditative experience using methodologies and perspectives that equally address the human condition and its search for truth.

MINDFULNESS IN MEDICAL EDUCATION AND PRACTICE

Medical training is a unique experience. Students and practitioners are expected to retain a vast amount of information and at the same time cultivate qualities of professionalism, which include compassion and empathy. Maintaining a balance between personal needs and the demands of medical training and practice is a balance many physicians neglect at the cost of their own well-being and health. Sleep, exercise, relaxation, and personal interests often take a back seat to long clinical hours and academic demands that contribute to burnout.[48]

Ironically, the medical learning environment can dampen the very characteristics it seeks to promote. Empathy, a core trait of quality medical care, is significantly diminished throughout medical school.[49] Stress, along with its many physical manifestations, is heightened throughout the many years of medical training and practice. It is troubling, therefore, to consider that cortisol, a biomarker of chronic stress, is implicated in diminished attention and memory function.[50] Research also shows that stress generates proinflammatory cytokines that have been directly linked with depression.[51]

Box 1
An example of getting started with mindfulness meditation practice: SOLAR (stop, observe, let it be, and return) and TIES (thought, image, emotion, and/or sensation)

STOP

- Find a quiet place where you will not be interrupted for the next several minutes.
- Set your cell phone alarm to vibrate in 5 or more minutes, and then forget about time altogether. You can adjust the length of your meditation time as you feel is appropriate.
- Sit comfortably in an alert position with a straight and relaxed back. With eyes open or closed, position your hands as you like.
- Allow an intention for this time, such as, "May I allow myself to be present to the simplicity of movements in the body as breathing, feeling, and sensing. May I enjoy the benefits of silence and stillness."

OBSERVE

- Direct your attention to noticing sensations in the body, noticing posture, feet on the floor, hips on the chair, or feeling a sense of being balanced and grounded.
- Allow the breath to flow in and out of the nose at a natural and unforced rate and depth. Avoid manipulating either a slower or a faster rate. Just let the body breathe. In your own bodily experience, notice the sensations of simply breathing.
- Moment by moment, allow yourself to take a pause, breathe, and feel exactly what arises in your experience.

LET IT BE

- For this time now let everything be as it is without reacting to or trying to change any of it. Like a watchful bystander, just witness your experience moment by moment as it happens right now, however it may be, pleasant or unpleasant.
- If you get caught up in any particular storyline, fantasy, daydream, rumination, compulsive thought, or distraction gently stop, drop into your body, and allow all experiences to roll on past the screen of your awareness like moving frames in a film.

AND...

RETURN

- Let the breath be your anchor in the present moment. If you get distracted or caught up in any particular TIES, just bring your attention back to the breath, returning repeatedly to the experience of breathing in a nonjudgemental and self-forgiving way.
- At the end of your meditation period, be still for a few more moments. Be aware of how you feel. Invite the intention to be mindfully present by taking a moment to pause, breathe, and feel whatever is happening in any experience throughout your day.

Box 2
Summary of mindfulness meditation practice

The experience (TIES mnemonic)

- Talk/thoughts: mental chatter, incessant thinking, storyline narratives
- Images: mental pictures, imagined scenes, visualized scenarios
- Emotions: love, hate, fear, joy, sadness, anxiety, and so on
- Physical sensations: sound, touch, sight, taste, smell

The process (SOLAR mnemonic)

- Stop: taking pause and dropping into this experience right now
- Observe: being aware of and noticing what is actually happening in this moment
- Let it be: acknowledging and allowing this arising experience to be what it is, pleasant or unpleasant
- And…
- Returning repeatedly to the present moment, remembering to pause, breathe, and feel whatever is happening

---

A 2009 study found the rate of depression in medical students to be 21.2%, more than double the rate for the general population.[52]

Mindfulness meditation addresses these concerns by offering a simple, yet effective tool to help ease many of the challenges, both personal and academic, encountered throughout medical training and practice. Medical students who participated in an 8-week MBSR course showed reduced anxiety, reduced distress and depression, and increased levels of empathy.[53] There is growing evidence that heightened

---

Box 3
Resources and links to learn meditation (links accessed 8 August 2009)

http://www.umassmed.edu/content.aspx?id=41252 (UMass Center for Mindfulness)

http://www.amsa.org/humed/ (AMSA Humanistic Medicine Group)

https://www.fammed.wisc.edu/aware-medicine/mindfulness (University of Wisconsin Aware Medicine Curriculum)

http://eomega.org/ (New York/east-coast Omega Institute)

http://nccam.nih.gov/ (NCCAM)

http://diydharma.org/about-us (Do It Yourself Dharma)

http://www.spiritrock.org/ (California/west-coast Meditation Center)

http://www.contemplativeoutreach.org/site/PageServer (Centering Prayer)

http://www.christinecenter.org (Wisconsin/mid-west Retreat Center)

Meditation for Beginners by Jack Kornfield PhD (book and CD)

Guided Mindfulness Meditation by Jon Kabat-Zinn (CD)

Full Catastrophe Living by Jon Kabat-Zinn (book)

Integrative Medicine, 2nd edition, edited by David Rakel, MD (Chapter 100 Recommending Meditation)

Open Mind Open Heart by Fr Thomas Keating OCSO (book)

The Beginner's Guide to Contemplative Prayer by James Finley PhD (CD)

Box 4
Precautions and recommendations for meditation practice

- Leg and back discomfort can be a common concern. Do not strain the body. Sit in an alert and comfortable position. Remember that meditation is about openness and not about contracting the body into discomfort.

- In the beginning, intrusive, repetitive, or disturbing thoughts may make it difficult to sit still for even 5 minutes. Keep in mind that meditation is not about making things go away. It is simply the nonjudgmental process of staying present with whatever is happening moment by moment, pleasant or unpleasant. However, over time with regular practice the mind will become more stable.

- In learning meditation, one should be guided by teachers and practices that resonate authentically, are nondivisive, and instill feelings of support. Do not forfeit personal boundaries and safety for any teacher or teaching. Listen to your intuition and reason, and trust that the experience you are having is exactly what you need in this moment.

- Meditation can at times uncover preexisting stressors or traumas, similar to peeling back the layers of an onion, revealing unpleasant underlying emotions. A professional counselor familiar with contemplative practice can help facilitate the healthy release of these emotions.

- Be attentive and honest with your experience. In a compassionate way, attend to realizations and insights that arise from regular meditation practice. This may include journaling, creative expression, and talking with a skilled meditation teacher.

- Including a gentle form of movement is encouraged, such as contemplative or mindful walking, walking the labyrinth, hatha yoga, pilates, nia, tai chi/qi gong, swimming, biking, etc. However, it is important to avoid striving and straining.

---

present-moment awareness gained through mindfulness training improves attention and memory.[54] Furthermore, Groopman[55] suggests that mindfulness meditation can help foster present-moment awareness that may reduce medical error and improve patient care. He asserts that faulty thinking such as snap judgments, distracted attention, inadvertent stereotyping, and other cognitive traps lead to critical mistakes in patient care, as opposed to the conventional understanding that medical errors are derived from lack of knowledge. These cognitive processing errors, which are not currently addressed in medical education, can be avoided by paying attention to the process of thinking by the metacognitive practice of mindfulness based self-reflection. Growing research also shows that practitioners who themselves exhibit healthy habits are more effective in motivating patients to make significant positive change in their life.[56] This is also true of health practitioners who practice meditation. In a randomized controlled trial of 124 psychiatric inpatients managed by 18 psychology residents, Grepmair and colleagues[57] showed that patients of interns who received mindfulness training did significantly better than those patients treated by interns who did not receive mindfulness training.

According to Astin and colleagues,[58] there is a strong need for more comprehensive training during medical school and residency for the application of mind-body methods such as meditation. There are a number of factors that help promote this. First, gaining the support of key administrative and academic leaders is crucial. Second, there should be an adequate and early introduction to self-reflective relaxation techniques in medical school, and recurrent opportunities to learn and practice meditation throughout medical training and practice (see **Boxes 1–3**). Third, it is important to acknowledge that student and practitioner populations are unique. Providing experientially based meditation teaching on a regular basis and reviewing current research will help practitioners and students better understand and skillfully use this mind-body tool personally and professionally. Finally, because it is difficult for anyone to incorporate a daily practice into his or her life (much less a stressed, sleep-deprived medical student or clinician) a responsive and pragmatic approach to meditation training in medicine is needed to address the specific needs of this time-limited professional demographic. **Boxes 1–3** offer some examples to help begin a mindful practice and opportunities for further training. **Box 4** offers recommendations and precautions to keep in mind when beginning to meditate.

SUMMARY

Meditation practice in the medical setting is proving to be an excellent adjunctive therapy for many illnesses and an essential and primary means of maintaining holistic health and wellness. Rather than being a fringe or marginal concept, meditation is now widely known and accepted as a beneficial mind-body practice by the general public and in the scientific community. Extensive research shows and continues to show the benefits of meditation practice for a wide range of medical conditions. Further efforts are required to operationalize and apply meditation practice in the clinical and medical educational settings in ways that are practical, effective, and meaningful.

ACKNOWLEDGMENTS

Special thanks to Katherine Bonus, MA, founder of the UW Health Mindfulness Program and Lisa R. Rambaldo, PsyD, founder of the Dean Medical System Mindfulness Services.

REFERENCES

1. Ludwig DS, Kabat-Zinn J. Mindfulness in medicine. JAMA 2008;300(11): 1350–2.
2. Deyo R, Mirza SK, Turner JA, et al. Overtreating chronic back pain, time to back off? J Am Board Fam Med 2009;22(1):62–8.
3. Paul-Labrador M, Polk D, Dwyer JH, et al. Effects of a randomized controlled trial of transcendental meditation on components of the metabolic syndrome in subjects with coronary heart disease. Arch Intern Med 2006;166(11): 1218–24.
4. McCray LW, Cronholm PF, Bogner HR, et al. Resident physician burnout, is there hope? Fam Med 2008;40(9):626–32.
5. Astin JA. Why patients use alternative medicine, results from a national study. JAMA 1998;279:1548–53.
6. Eckleberry-Hunt J, Lick D, Boura J, et al. An exploratory study of resident burnout and wellness. Acad Med 2009;84(2):269–77.
7. Chiesa A, Serretti A. Mindfulness based stress reduction for stress management in healthy people, a review and meta-analysis. J Altern Complement Med 2009; 15(5):593–600.
8. Lerner M. Choice in cancer—integrating the best of conventional and alternative approaches to cancer. Cambridge (MA): MIT Press; 1994.
9. Beck CJ. Everyday zen. New York: HarperCollins; 1989.
10. Brosse T. A psychophysiological study. Main Current Mod Thought 1946;4:77–84.
11. Wenger MA, Bagchi BK. Studies of autonomic functions in practitioners of yoga in India. Behav Sci 1961;6:312–23.

12. Vakil R. Remarkable feat of endurance of a yogi priest. Lancet 1950;2:871.
13. Hoenig J. Medical research on yoga. Confin Psychiatr 1968;11:69–89.
14. La Rovere MT, Bigger JT Jr, Marcus FI, et al. Baroreflex sensitivity and heart-rate variability in prediction of total cardiac mortality after myocardial infarction. Lancet 1998;351:478–84.
15. Nolan J, Batin PD, Andrews R, et al. Prospective study of heart rate variability and mortality in chronic heart failure—results of the United Kingdom heart failure evaluation and assessment of risk trial. Circulation 1998;98:1510–6.
16. Bernardi L, Sleight P, Bandinelli G, et al. Effect of rosary prayer and yoga mantras on autonomic cardiovascular rhythms—comparative study. BMJ 2001;323:1446–9.
17. Peng CK, Henry IC, Mietus JE, et al. Heart rate dynamics during three forms of meditation. Int J Cardiol 2004;95(1):19–27.
18. Benson H, Kotch JB, Crassweller KD. The relaxation response—a bridge between psychiatry and medicine. Med Clin North Am 1977;61:929–38.
19. Kabat-Zinn J, Massion AO, Kristeller J, et al. Effectiveness of a mindfulness-based stress reduction program in the treatment of anxiety disorders. Am J Psychiatry 1992;149(7):936–43.
20. Miller J, Fletcher K, Kabat-Zinn J. Three-year follow-up and clinical implications of a mindfulness meditation-based stress reduction intervention in the treatment of anxiety disorders. Gen Hosp Psychiatry 1995;17(3):192–200.
21. Beauchamp-Turner D, Levinson D. Effects of meditation on stress, health, and affect. Medical-Psychother Int J 1992;5:123–31.
22. Teasdale J, Segal ZV, Williams JM, et al. Prevention of relapse/recurrence in major depression by mindfulness-based cognitive therapy. J Consult Clin Psychol 2000;68(4):615–23.
23. Ma SH, Teasdale JD. Mindfulness-based cognitive therapy for depression—replication and exploration of differential relapse prevention effects. J Consult Clin Psychol 2004;72(1):31–40.
24. Kabat-Zinn J, Lipworth L, Burney R. The clinical use of mindfulness meditation for the self-regulation of chronic pain. J Behav Med 1985;8(2):163–90.
25. Blanchard EB, Nicholson NL, Taylor AE, et al. The role of regular home practice in the relaxation treatment of tension headache. J Consult Clin Psychol 1991;59:467–70.
26. Kabat-Zinn J, Wheeler E, Light T, et al. Influence of a mindfulness-based stress reduction intervention on rates of skin clearing in patients with moderate to severe psoriasis undergoing phototherapy and photochemotherapy. Psychosom Med 1998;60:625–32.
27. Alexander CN, Schneider RH, Staggers F, et al. Trial of stress reduction for hypertension in older African Americans. Hypertension 1996;28:228–37.
28. Parati G, Steptoe A. Stress reduction and blood pressure control in hypertension—a role for transcendental meditation? J Hypertens 2004;22(11):2057–60.
29. Cooper M, Aygen M. Effect of meditation on blood cholesterol and blood pressure. Harefuah 1978;95(1):1–2.
30. Royer-Bounour P. The transcendental meditation technique—a new direction for smoking cessation programs. Abstr Int 1989;50(8):3428B.
31. Davis JM, Fleming MF, Bonus KA, et al. A pilot study on mindfulness based stress reduction for smokers. BMC Complement Altern Med 2007;25:2–7.
32. Zgierska A, Rabago D, Zuelsdorff M, et al. Mindfulness meditation for alcohol relapse prevention, a feasibility pilot study. J Addict Med 2008;2(3):165–73.
33. Fields JZ, Walton KG, Schneider RH, et al. Effect of a multimodality natural medicine program on carotid atherosclerosis in older subjects—a pilot trial of Maharishi Vedic Medicine. Am J Cardiol 2002;89:952–8.

34. Zamarra JW, Schneider RH, Besseghini I, et al. Usefulness of the transcendental meditation program in the treatment of patients with coronary artery disease. Am J Cardiol 1996;77:867–70.

35. Ornish D, Brown SE, Scherwitz LW, et al. Can lifestyle changes reverse coronary heart disease? Lancet 1990;336:129–33.

36. Alexander CN, Langer EJ, Newman RI, et al. Transcendental meditation, mindfulness, and longevity—an experimental study with the elderly. J Pers Soc Psychol 1989;57:950–64.

37. Shannahoff-Khalsa D. An introduction to kundalini yoga meditation techniques that are specific for the treatment of psychiatric disorders. J Altern Complement Med 2004;10(1):91–101.

38. Shearer S, Gordon L. The patient with excessive worry. Am Fam Physician 2006; 73(6):1049–56.

39. Orme-Johnson D. Medical care utilization and the transcendental meditation program. Psychosom Med 1987;49:493–507.

40. Caudill M, Schnable R, Zuttermeister P, et al. Decreased clinic use by chronic pain patients—response to behavioral medicine intervention. Clin J Pain 1991; 7:305–10.

41. Grossman P, Niemann L, Schmidt S, et al. Mindfulness-based stress reduction and health benefits—a meta-analysis. J Psychosom Res 2004;57:35–43.

42. Newberg AB, Iversen J. The neural basis of the complex mental task of meditation—neurotransmitter and neurochemical considerations. Med Hypotheses 2003;61(2):282–91.

43. Davidson RJ, Kabat-Zinn J, Schumacher J, et al. Alterations in brain and immune function produced by mindfulness meditation. Psychosom Med 2003;65:564–70.

44. Hayney MS, Love GD, Buck JM, et al. The association between psychosocial factors and vaccine-induced cytokine production. Vaccine 2003;21: 2428–32.

45. Rosenkranz MA, Jackson DC, Dalton KM, et al. Affective style and in vivo immune response—neurobehavioral mechanisms. Proc Natl Acad Sci U S A 2003; 100(19):11148–52.

46. Cohen S, Herbert TB. Health psychology—psychological factors and physical disease from the perspective of human psychoneuroimmunology. Annu Rev Psychol 1996;47:113–42.

47. Lutz A, Greischar LL, Rawlings NB, et al. Long-term meditators self-induce high-amplitude gamma synchrony during mental practice. Proc Natl Acad Sci U S A 2004;101(46):16369–73.

48. Dyrbye LN, Thomas MR, Massie FS, et al. Burnout and suicidal ideation among US medical students. Ann Intern Med 2008;149:334–41.

49. Newton B, Barber L, Clardy J, et al. Is there a hardening of the heart during medical school? Acad Med 2008;83:244–9.

50. Newcomer J, Selke G, Melson A, et al. Decreased memory performance in healthy humans induced by stress-level cortisol treatment. Arch Gen Psychiatry 1999;56:527–33.

51. Dowlati Y, Herrmann N, Swardfager W, et al. A meta-analysis of cytokines in major depression. Biol Psychiatry 2009, in press.

52. Goebert D, Thompson D, Takeshita J, et al. Depressive symptoms in medical students and residents: a multischool study. Acad Med 2009;84:236–41.

53. Shapiro S, Schwartz G, Bonner G. Effects of mindfulness-based stress reduction on medical and premedical students. J Behav Med 1998;21:581–99.

54. Jha A, Krompinger J, Baime M. Mindfulness training modifies subsystems of attention. Cogn Affect Behav Neurosci 2007;7(2):109–19.
55. Groopman J. How doctors think. Boston: Houghton Mifflin; 2007.
56. Frank E, Breyan J, Elon L. Physician disclosure of healthy personal behaviors improves credibility and ability to motivate. Arch Fam Med 2000;9:287–90.
57. Grepmair L, Mitterlehner F, Loew T, et al. Promoting mindfulness in psychotherapists in training influences the treatment results of their patients, a randomized double blind controlled study. Psychother Psychosom 2007;76:332–8.
58. Astin JA, Sierpina VS, Forys K, et al. Integration of the biopsychosocial model, perspectives of medical students and residents. Acad Med 2008;83:20–7.

Biofeedback and Primary Care

Ronald M. Glick, MD[a,b,*], Carol M. Greco, PhD[b]

KEYWORDS

- Biofeedback • Neurofeedback
- Integrative medicine • Mind–body

Biofeedback is defined as a process that enables an individual to learn how to change physiologic activity for the purposes of improving health and performance. Precise instruments measure physiologic activity such as brainwaves, heart function, breathing, muscle activity, and skin temperature. These instruments rapidly and accurately feed back information to the user. The presentation of this information—often in conjunction with changes in thinking, emotions, and behavior—supports desired physiologic changes. Over time, these changes can endure without continued use of an instrument.[29]

The most prominent use of biofeedback is to train individuals in physiologic relaxation and stress reduction. It long has been known that yogis and others who practice eastern mind–body techniques can induce a state of relaxation sufficient to greatly slow their heart rate and influence other autonomic processes. Since the 1950s, the technology has become available to allow individuals to attain similar physiologic states that previously had been assumed to be outside of conscious control. In tandem with this development, knowledge of the physiologic stress response has increased greatly over the last several decades. Combining the research knowledge of the physiologic changes associated with stressful situations together with learning theory, psychologists employed the available technology (eg, EMG) to allow patients to observe and learn to change their stress response patterns. Over the last 30 years, there has been a dramatic growth in the use of biofeedback, in terms of forms of feedback used, conditions that may be treated, and clinical trials research supporting the efficacy of treatment.[30] There are an estimated 1500 certified biofeedback practitioners in the United States and a recent survey of usage of complementary therapies found a doubling from 0.1% of adults in 2002 to 0.2% in 2007 who reported using biofeedback during the previous year.[31]

[a] Department of Psychiatry, Physical Medicine and Rehabilitation, and Family Medicine, University of Pittsburgh School of Medicine, 580 South Aiken Suite 310, Pittsburgh, PA 15232, USA
[b] Department of Psychiatry, University of Pittsburgh School of Medicine, Center for Integrative Medicine at UPMC Shadyside, 580 South Aiken Suite 310, Pittsburgh, PA 15232, USA
* Corresponding author.
E-mail address: glickrm@upmc.edu (R.M. Glick).

Prim Care Clin Office Pract 37 (2010) 91–103
doi:10.1016/j.pop.2009.09.005
0095-4543/10/$ – see front matter © 2010 Elsevier Inc. All rights reserved.

Key Points	Evidence Level	Reference
Anxiety disorders and insomnia (modulating stress response is central to many indications for biofeedback); strongest support is for neurofeedback	B	1,2
Headaches—multiple well-designed studies have confirmed benefit for both tension-type and migraine headaches	A	3,4
Abdominal pain and functional gastrointestinal (GI) disorders—despite wide clinical use, literature reports are primarily anecdotal	C	5
Low back pain, neck pain, myofascial pain	B	6,7
Fibromyalgia	B	8–10
Temporomandibular joint dysfunction	A	11
Attention-deficit/hyperactivity disorder (ADHD)—neurofeedback is seen as having a moderate effect on attention and behavior	A	12,13
Urinary incontinence—there is strong evidence for benefit of electromyogram (EMG) biofeedback	A	14
Seizures—as noted in the text, two specific approaches appear promising	B	15
Coronary heart disease and hypertension	B	2,16–20
Chronic obstructive pulmonary disease (COPD) and asthma	B	21–23
Pelvic pain	B	24
Raynaud syndrome	B	25
Fecal incontinence and constipation	B	26–28

If the goal of biofeedback is simply to induce a relaxation response, why should not one just employ other behavioral and mind–body techniques instead? First, as will be noted, biofeedback may be of benefit for many conditions other than those directly associated with stress. To the extent that many of the problems for which biofeedback is used may have a psychological component, it is reasonable to offer other approaches such as progressive muscle relaxation (PMR), mindfulness meditation, yoga, and guided imagery. In fact, psychologists often use other mind–body techniques coupled with biofeedback, and they may employ cognitive behavioral or other psychotherapeutic strategies also.

The continuum between a stress response and relaxation state can be described in terms of the sympathovagal balance of the autonomic nervous system.[32] Many of the chronic conditions seen in primary care display a sympathetic predominant pattern, including: anxiety disorders, depression, chronic pain states, coronary artery disease, hypertension, and diabetes. Will shifting this balance result in clinical improvement? The efficacy of beta-blockers following acute myocardial infarction is one example of how modifying adrenergic tone may be beneficial. Although a great antistress pill is not available, simple behavioral techniques coupled with biofeedback can reliably result in the same beneficial changes.

When one is in an acute stressful situation, either an external event or an internally driven sense of threat, several physiologic changes occur. One may be aware of one's heart racing and palms becoming sweaty. Another change of which one is often less aware of is coolness of the extremities, brought on by peripheral vasoconstriction. Increased muscle tension often is reported during stress. In particular, patients with headache or back pain frequently note muscles tightening up in stressful situations. Other changes are less available to conscious awareness, such as a shift in electroencephalogram (EEG) pattern and a decrease in heart rate variability (HRV). Essentially, if one can measure it, one can use biofeedback to gain awareness of the pattern and learn to change it. There are some autonomic changes seen with stress, however, including blood pressure or pupillary response, that can be measured but for which direct biofeedback applications are not currently employed. Because the stress response is a set of related physiologic processes, intervention using one or two forms of biofeedback should result in reduction in arousal of the entire system. For example EMG and peripheral temperature (thermal) biofeedback may help a patient learn to relax muscles and dilate peripheral blood vessels. Blood pressure, breathing rate, and heart rate are likely to show corresponding changes.

FORMS OF BIOFEEDBACK

The following is a list of some of the most commonly used forms of biofeedback:

EMG—surface electrodes are applied to specific muscles with the intensity of muscle activity reflected in the amplitude of signal. This is used most commonly in pain conditions such as low back or other myofascial pain states, tension-type headaches, and anxiety disorders. Other uses include muscle retraining following stroke or other nerve injury and pelvic floor and continence dysfunction. For most conditions, the goal is to learn to let go of muscle tension, but for motor retraining, the goal is improve the conscious activation of muscles.

Thermal—a skin probe is placed, typically on a finger, with the patient guided to engage in relaxation activities that will help warm the hand or increase temperature. Just as stress can induce cooling of the extremities, learning to warm the hands tends to lead to a relaxation response. Given the observation of cerebral vasodilatation in migraine, it is hypothesized that increasing peripheral circulation may attenuate the headache, although the relaxation response is likely equally important.

Electrodermal (also referred to as galvanic skin response or GSR feedback)—electrical probes are placed on the skin, typically the palmar surface of the fingers. The electrical conductance between the two probes is related directly to the amount of sweat secreted, with resistance being the reciprocal of this. The patient learns how to decrease the level of conductance displayed. This is another technique that can be helpful for pain and anxiety states.

Neurofeedback (or EEG biofeedback)—this is derived from the advances in neurology and psychiatry with the study of quantitative EEG (QEEG). Fourier analysis of the raw EEG signal allows the breakdown of the irregular waveforms into a determination of the prominent frequency patterns. Specific EEG patterns may be present in conditions such as ADHD, Asperger syndrome, and epilepsy. Through biofeedback training, individuals can learn to shift the predominant frequencies to a level deemed beneficial for the condition being treated.

HRV biofeedback—this involves the use of a photoplethysmography probe placed on the index finger or ear lobe, which detects the flushing of the skin that occurs with each cardiac contraction. The screen displays the moment-to-moment heart rate, similar to what might read out on a cardiac monitor. A computer algorithm analyzes the frequency pattern and provides visual and auditory feedback to facilitate a pattern associated with a relaxed and focused state. This approach has potential indications for anxiety- and stress-related problems, respiratory problems such as asthma and COPD, hypertension, and cardiac arrhythmia. HRV biofeedback takes advantage of the physiologic phenomenon of respiratory sinus arrhythmia (RSA), which one observes every day in chest auscultation, with inspiration increasing the heart rate slightly and expiration resulting in cardiac slowing. Through paced breathing and use of imagery techniques, the plot of heart rate over time shows a coherent pattern, in which a smooth sinusoidal pattern is seen and one can predict from moment to moment if the heart rate is likely to accelerate or decelerate. This is in contrast to the chaotic pattern one typically exhibits during a crazy, busy, multitasking day, in which the amplitude of the fluctuation in heart rate is decreased, and the up and down variation appears totally random. The coherent picture reflects parasympathetic predominance, and the more irregular or chaotic pattern is associated with withdrawal of parasympathetic and increased sympathetic activity.

TECHNOLOGICAL AND PRACTICAL CONSIDERATIONS

Given the progress in the computer gaming industry, tremendous strides are occurring in the quality of the visual and auditory displays used in biofeedback applications. Amazing software geared toward children and adolescents has been developed, in which success at games is tied to implementing the relaxation response. Similar to the phenomenon of parents hogging their kids' X-Box, adults often find these games more intriguing and motivating than the simple auditory and visual output displays historically used for biofeedback training. Typically, the biofeedback instrumentation is used within a session, and the patient is instructed to go home and practice the appropriate relaxation techniques without the use of technology. This has the advantage of fostering a sense of competence and self-efficacy outside of the biofeedback suite. Technology strikes again, however. Inexpensive portable home units are available for daily practice, particularly with HRV biofeedback.

GOALS OF BIOFEEDBACK

Regardless of the modality of biofeedback or the condition being treated, there are similar goals for a course of treatment. The general goals and aims include:

1. Education regarding the connections between the patient's symptoms and his or her physiology;
2. Specific skills training in changing the auditory or visual biofeedback signals corresponding to physiologic processes;
3. Development of awareness of the internal states that are linked to the arousal and relaxation;
4. Application of the skills training to include carry-over in recognizing and modifying internal states without the aid of instrumentation;
5. Development of an overall sense of self-efficacy and empowerment for contributing to health and well being, regardless of the extent to which the presenting problem has been resolved.

Biofeedback procedures can be particularly helpful for patients with chronic or disabling conditions. It is common for these patients to be frustrated and angry. Often, they have relied on the medical system only to find that expectations for a cure or significant relief of symptoms have not been met. Another concern is that these patients may assume a passive role, feel helpless and hopeless, and have limited sense of control or self-efficacy regarding their condition. Finally, it is not unusual for individuals with these conditions to have comorbid psychiatric disorders, particularly in the anxiety and depression spectra. Consequently, health care providers may identify goals that are slightly different than the patients' primary concern. Obviously, from the patients' perspective the main objective is to eliminate or greatly minimize the pain or symptoms. The first challenge for the biofeedback practitioner is to help the patient think not in terms of all or none, but to recognize any progress as steps toward their goals.

Although the novelty of biofeedback may place it on a par with hypnosis and acupuncture as somehow magical, another goal is to help patients view themselves as the agent for change and recognize that improvement is the result of one's own behaviors and attitudes as much as, or even more than, any medical intervention. Regarding associated anxiety and depression, while these may require specific treatment approaches, by engaging in the biofeedback process and practicing the skills at home, patients often describe greater control over anxiety symptoms and a sense of hopefulness and purpose. These cognitive shifts could be considered as part of a cognitive–behavioral therapy (CBT) approach, but they are part and parcel of the treatment provided by a skilled biofeedback practitioner.

Although it is possible to accomplish physiologic change with other behavioral medicine or mind–body approaches that do not use instrumentation, a potential advantage of the biofeedback approach is acceptability. Patients with chronic conditions, particularly pain, often perceive physicians or friends as suggesting that their problems are primarily psychological. Consequently, it is not surprising to find that they are resistant to the idea of a psychological or psychiatric consultation, and many patients decline the referral for that reason. Although physicians are aware of the psychosomatic connection, from a patient's perspective, the focus on physiologic changes makes biofeedback a more palatable treatment. Although the agenda is purportedly working on these physical phenomena, biofeedback can give a back door into addressing a stress-related component and engaging the patient in self-management strategies.

Another obstacle to a more traditional psychotherapeutic approach occurs when the patient is seen as not psychologically minded, having difficulty articulating affective experiences or exploring the effect of life stressors on mood, anxiety, and physical symptoms. Biofeedback can be a hook to draw such patients into the partnership of treatment by illustrating visually how stress imagery or the practice of relaxation techniques such as rhythmic breathing influence physiologic markers. Some patients, particularly those with more of a left-brain orientation, are drawn to the technological aspects of biofeedback, and this can enhance motivation to participate in this modality of treatment.

PROCESS OF TREATMENT

Although the treatment protocol is different for each modality, particularly for specialized areas such as neurofeedback and treatment of pelvic floor dysfunction, there are some commonalities to the structure and approach of a course of treatment of biofeedback.

Initial Session

As with any other medical encounter, initially the clinician performs an evaluation. Typically, this involves an assessment of the patient's perception of the problem, including etiology, provocative and palliative factors, and impact on functioning. Additionally, it is important to assess psychological functioning and coping strategies and screen for psychiatric disorders that might require specific treatment. Similar to any therapeutic relationships, making a connection with the patient and conveying a sense of purpose and hope for change are essential ingredients.

When moving into the biofeedback itself, it is important to provide a plausible rationale for the treatment, and it is most helpful if the rationale is presented in a way that is congruent with the patient's perception of problems. For example a headache sufferer who sees no connection with stress and headaches might be presented with an explanation about the role of cerebral vasodilatation in the etiology of migraines with the idea that by warming the hands one might attenuate the pathologic process. In this case, the importance of the explanation is to get buy-in on the part of the patient.

In the initial session, once patients are connected to the biofeedback equipment, it is helpful to allow them to see the initial level of activity of whatever is being measured (eg, trapezius muscle tone on EMG). At that point, one could engage the patient in imagery of a stressful situation to illustrate the impact of stress on physiology. Next, the biofeedback therapist may guide the patient in a relaxation exercise (eg, paced breathing). At this stage, it is very important to create a success-oriented atmosphere, and minimize the potential that the patient interprets less-than-optimal ability to change biofeedback signals as failure. This can be accomplished by starting the training with the biofeedback sensors detached. Once the patient develops some confidence, and the clinician observes signs of physiologic change, such as slowed respiration, the therapist may connect sensors. When the patient has observed the change in physiology with the behavioral intervention, the final task is to assign the practice of the activity (eg, paced breathing) at home. At this point, the goals of the 1st session have been accomplished: the assessment is completed, a therapeutic relationship is being formed, a plausible rationale has been presented, the patient has been engaged in treatment, and the patient has accepted the responsibility for practicing. **Fig. 1** provides photos of a typical session, and **Fig. 2** shows a close-up of a biofeedback computer display.

Subsequent Sessions

Subsequent sessions involve processing how the practice has gone and observations as far as change in symptoms or any other changes noted. For pain and stress-related conditions, the initial goal is to engage the patient in regular daily practice of activities that were effective in changing their physiologic responses during the sessions. Typically, with each session, the patient accomplishes the changes more quickly. Autogenic (self-statements regarding capability to make appropriate changes [eg, in hand temperature]) and relaxation activities can be varied to find what works the best for the patient. Similarly, the modality of biofeedback can be changed

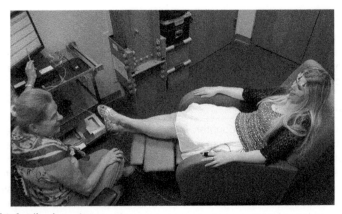

Fig. 1. A biofeedback session.

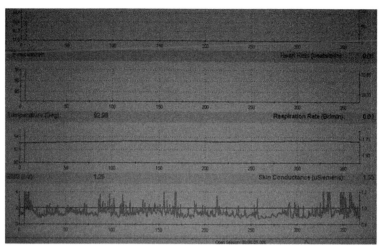

Fig. 2. Example of a computer display from a biofeedback session.

(eg, from thermal to EMG for someone with a mixed migraine- and tension-type head-ache picture). For episodic conditions such as abdominal pain or migraines, as the treatment progresses, it is important to extend the activities from daily practice to employing the relaxation activities during the event (eg, visualization to warm hands during a migraine aura). Gradually, over a course of treatment, there is less of an emphasis on the biofeedback and more on self-practice.

As the sessions progress, patients typically become their own biofeedback device. They learn to recognize internal states of hyperarousal or stress reactivity without the assistance of the biofeedback machinery. In fact, often the patient becomes adept at recognizing even small or early cues of overarousal. Having learned the process of decreasing this arousal, the patient can implement the relaxation response in any setting, although some settings or situations may be quite challenging. The patient's efforts toward reducing arousal may be rewarded both internally and externally. The internal reward may manifest as pain reduction, a greater sense of calm, or a sense of mastery and self-efficacy. External reinforcement may take the form of decreased irritability and greater ease and connection in interpersonal relationships.

CLINICAL CONDITIONS

Although it is impossible to provide an exhaustive list of all conditions treated with biofeedback, here is included a sampling of topics of potential interest to the primary care physician. Some have a solid track record in clinical trials, while others are included given the prevalence of the conditions, the associated morbidity or distress, and the potential for biofeedback to be of benefit. The following disorders share many characteristics:

1. They are prevalent in the general population and primary care practice.
2. They result in significant functional impairment or impact on quality of life.
3. They often respond only partially to traditional medical treatment approaches.

Anxiety Disorders and Insomnia

The most frequent reason for using biofeedback is to help a person with conditions related to sympathetic hyperarousal learn to have greater awareness of their physiologic state and learn techniques to turn that around. EMG, thermal, electrodermal, and neurofeedback all have been used successfully for anxiety disorders. Despite the widespread clinical use, only a moderate body of research exists. Neurofeedback has been studied most, with findings of excellent reduction in self-report of symptoms and a moderate change in EEG pattern with increase in alpha rhythms.[1] Additionally, some studies support the benefit of EMG and neurofeedback for insomnia, but given the limited data, it would be reasonable to include this as an additional self-management strategy in a course of CBT.

Headaches

The strongest evidence for the benefit of biofeedback lies in the treatment of migraines and tension-type headaches, with studies in both adults and children. These conditions are among the most common reasons for referrals to biofeedback clinicians. A recent meta-analysis and systematic review of over 100 studies showed a moderate reduction of headache symptoms for both of these headache conditions.[3] Given the strength of the evidence, biofeedback for headache is considered an established medical treatment, with many headache clinics having in-house or community resources available.[4] Because of the vascular etiology of migraine, thermal biofeedback has been studied most frequently. Similarly, given the common impression of muscle tension as contributing to tension-type headache, EMG biofeedback has been used most commonly for this condition. In practice, the boundaries blur for three reasons:

1. It is quite common to have a mixed headache picture.
2. Both thermal and EMG biofeedback modalities share the effect of decreasing sympathetic activity and inducing a relaxation response.
3. Regardless of the etiology, some patients respond to one modality of biofeedback better than another.

Abdominal Pain and Functional GI Disorders

Common functional GI disorders include irritable bowel syndrome, functional dyspepsia, and recurrent abdominal pain of childhood. As with other chronic pain conditions, these may have a strong psychological component, and patients often describe becoming aware that they are stressed following the development of GI symptoms. Various mind–body approaches have shown benefit for these conditions, particularly hypnotherapy. Only a few studies have addressed biofeedback for abdominal pain and GI disorders, and the research design of these studies was only fair rather than optimal.[5] This is in contrast to the frequency of referral from primary physicians and gastroenterologists for biofeedback and the excellent response that is seen anecdotally in clinical practice. Consequently, one is left with a potentially useful intervention for chronic and disabling conditions, with only limited clinical trials supporting efficacy. As with other complementary modalities, patients are less concerned about randomized controlled trials than the clinician's expectations that a treatment likely will offer relief of symptoms.

Low Back Pain, Neck Pain, Tempromandibular Joint Dysfunction, Myofascial Pain, and Fibromyalgia

Although these conditions often have mixed etiologies, there appears to be a common denominator of tight muscles potentially contributing to pain. Considerations for treatment of tight muscles include:

Muscle relaxants—which are associated with sedation
Injections—which are somewhat invasive
Stretching techniques—which should be used in conjunction with any other
  intervention
Mind–body approaches.

Biofeedback has the unique advantage of providing the patient with direct information as to how tight or loose specific muscle groups are, also giving immediate feedback regarding the impact of stress-related imagery versus relaxation techniques on
the muscle tone. Several studies conducted in the 1980s and 1990s showed promise
for this modality for myofascial pain syndromes and low back pain, but this work has
not been replicated in recent years.[6,7] Temporomandibular joint disorders have been
studied most extensively, with a moderate level of support for the use of EMG biofeedback.[11] Several studies of fibromyalgia have found improvement in pain, quality of life,
and psychological distress. Modalities employed have included EMG and HRV feedback, as well as neurofeedback.[8–10]

ADHD

Given the observation that individuals with ADHD have a prominent theta (slow wave)
pattern to their EEG during periods when they should be attending to tasks, programs
have been developed to provide favorable feedback (eg, progress in a game) when
a patient increases the beta activity and decreases theta.[12,13] When EMG biofeedback
is used, the signal may relate to something in a patient's everyday experience, such as
tightening a muscle. Neurofeedback is less intuitive, but nonetheless, children and
adolescents seem to learn quickly how to shift the balance of their EEG pattern.
The protocols established have found clinically and statistically significant improvement in attention, socialization, and behavioral control, but they require upwards of
40 sessions to accomplish these gains. The benefits can be lasting and result in
some sparing of stimulant medication, which is often part of the parents' motivation
when seeking unconventional treatments.[33]

Urinary Incontinence

Particularly for postmenopausal women, urinary incontinence (UI) is quite an exasper-
ating problem, often with limited response to medications available. In general, EMG
biofeedback can be used to help strengthen weak muscles and increase awareness of
tight muscles. Specific to UI, treatment most commonly is directed to incompetence
of the pelvic floor muscles (PFM), particularly the levator ani, but treatment also can be
used for overactivity of the detrusor.[14] A small probe, the size and shape of a tampon,
is placed in the vagina. By increasing awareness of the PFM tone, the patient learns to
increase activation of these muscles. With improved awareness of the muscle activity
and increased voluntary control, patients are commonly able to decrease episodes of
urgency and incontinence after a short series of sessions, coupled with home practice.
As opposed to other forms of biofeedback, which generally are the domain of psychologists, treatment of pelvic pain and UI is provided commonly by physical therapists
who have undergone specialized training in women's health and pelvic floor problems.

Seizures

The common understanding of seizures suggests that these are random events that
are beyond voluntary control. The inference is that biofeedback would be unlikely to
be of benefit. For most individuals, seizures are controlled with medication, and no
further intervention is necessary. There are many patients, however, in any

neurologist's practice, who continue to break through with some seizures despite receiving multiple anticonvulsant medications. As noted previously, neurofeedback can be used to make a person aware of the dominant frequency of their EEG signal and learn to change that pattern. Sensorimotor rhythm (SMR), in which EEG activity is between 12 and 14 Hz, appears to have a preventive effect, reducing the likelihood of seizures. Sterman[15] provides a useful summary of the scientific rationale and experimental background, with the original finding that cats could be trained to produce this SMR and reduce the likelihood of seizures, leading to the development of this currently used neurofeedback protocol. A second finding is that negative slow cortical potentials (SCP) (<1 Hz) often occur before a seizure episode. Consequently, another approach is feedback to decrease negative SCP and increase positive SCP.

Coronary Heart Disease and Hypertension

HRV is a marker of risk for heart disease. Compared with cardiac patients with a normal level of HRV, particularly the high-frequency (HF) component, those with decreased HRV have an increased risk of cardiac events or sudden death, with an odds ratio of 2 or greater.[16,17] To some extent, decreased HRV is likely a marker of more severe heart disease, reflecting decreased ability on the part of the cardiovascular system to modify its output in response to demands. Additionally, decreased HRV may be an indication of prominence of sympathetic activity and decreased parasympathetic control of the heart. Biofeedback can impact on this phenomenon directly, fostering a decrease in sympathetic influence and increase in parasympathetic influence.[19] One form of biofeedback, which ties in directly with the respiratory pattern with a proprietary device (RESPeRATE), has resulted in a significant reduction in blood pressure among hypertensive patients.[18,20] Similarly, HRV biofeedback, which also takes advantage of respiratory patterns, can be helpful for managing hypertension. Two major bodies of practice and research have led to protocols in use, and although they are described for heart disease, the applications of this approach are much wider. The Institute of HeartMath has developed therapy protocols that couple the relaxed and alert states of coherence, as described previously, along with positive emotional experiences. Studies by McCraty[2,34] have shown a decrease in blood pressure and improvement in psychological outcomes both in healthy patients and individuals with hypertension. A second group, with studies by Lehrer and others, has focused on the idea of a resonant frequency.[35] This is based on the understanding that different components of HRV are associated with different physiologic phenomena. A large component of HRV is determined by respiratory sinus arrhythmia (RSA), which is generally in the range of 0.15 to 0.4 Hz. A second component of HRV is associated with an inherent baroreceptor reflex, which is generally around 0.08 to 0.1 Hz. If one slows respirations down to 6 breaths per minute or slightly less, the RSA and baroreceptor components of HRV overlap or resonate, leading to a profound shift to parasympathetic predominance. By varying respiratory rate during the biofeedback session, one can determine the number of breaths per minute that results in this resonant pattern. Typically, it is in the range of 6 breaths per minute for an average adult—slightly lower for males, those physically fit, and individuals who engage in regular mind-body practice. The number of breaths per minute resulting in resonant frequency is slightly higher for children.

Other Conditions that May Benefit from Biofeedback

Studies have supported clinical improvements with biofeedback for asthma and COPD,[21–23] Raynaud's syndrome,[25] chronic pelvic pain,[24] fecal incontinence,[28] and chronic constipation.[26,27] Other conditions with a psychosomatic component such as chronic itching and dermatitis may benefit also.

RESEARCH ISSUES

As with other psychotherapy techniques and complementary therapies, a major concern in the biofeedback literature is the choice of control or comparison group. The most commonly used control is a wait list or nontreatment group, which controls for time but not treatment expectation. A novel approach is to use bogus feedback, in which the visual or auditory display, which supposedly provides information about the subject's physiologic state, instead provides random feedback.

INSURANCE AND REIMBURSEMENT ISSUES

There are standard current procedural terminology (CPT) codes for biofeedback, and these should be recognized by major health insurance plans. Consequently, one would expect that biofeedback would be covered universally by third-party payers. Unfortunately, several factors may limit the reimbursement available to consumers. Some insurers may limit coverage for biofeedback and health and behavior codes. Additionally, reimbursement by psychologists and other therapists may be covered by the mental health component of health insurance plans, which may necessitate diagnosis of a primary psychiatric disorder, which may be at odds with a patient's perception that the problem (eg, migraines) is primarily physical. Finally, in many communities, the biofeedback-trained clinicians may operate on a cash basis. Patients can seek reimbursement from their insurers for out-of-network coverage.

TRAINING AND CREDENTIALING

Most commonly, practitioners of biofeedback already are trained in clinical psychology or another mental health discipline. This background has the advantage that the clinician is likely to be familiar with the general approach of evaluation and goal-directed treatment and should be comfortable with the possibility that a benign intervention may bring up disquieting emotional issues with the patient. Practitioners also come from medicine, nursing, physical therapy, and other health-related disciplines. The training typically involves initial conferences or seminars and accompanied reading to learn the theoretical background and basic practical approaches.

Subsequently, it is important to experience a course of biofeedback—either for general relaxation and wellness, or for a specific problem such as migraines or neck and shoulder pain. When one begins treating patients, it is important to work with a mentor or supervisor who can provide appropriate clinical supervision. The Association for Psychophysiology and Applied Biofeedback and the Biofeedback Certification Institute of America (BCIA) provide the structure and guidelines for this training and certification. When looking for potential resources in the community, if a practitioner has gone through the BCIA credentialing process, the referring physician can be confident that there has been a reasonable standard of training.

RESOURCES

Organizations include:

> *Association for Psychophysiology and Applied Biofeedback* is an organization involved in promoting research, clinical practice, and education related to biofeedback (http://www.aapb.org/home.html). *BCIA* is the central body that

provides credentialing for biofeedback practitioners. This organization provides a directory of certified practitioners http://www.bcia.org/.

The Institute of HeartMath is an organization that has developed PC-based and hand-held HRV biofeedback programs as well as a therapy approach for stress management, and the organization engages in training and research. This organization also has sponsored several research studies, has several publications describing its approach, and provides training http://www.heartmath.org/.

The best single reference for the initiated is *Biofeedback—A Practioner's Guide*, 3rd edition, by Mark Schwartz and published by Guilford Press.

REFERENCES

1. Hammond DC. Neurofeedback with anxiety and affective disorders. Child Adolesc Psychiatr Clin N Am 2005;14:105–23, vii.
2. McCraty R, Atkinson M, Tomasino D, et al. Impact of a workplace stress reduction program on blood pressure and emotional health in hypertensive employees. J Altern Complement Med 2003;9:355–69.
3. Nestoriuc Y, Martin A, Nestoriuc Y, et al. Efficacy of biofeedback for migraine: a meta-analysis. Pain 2007;128:111–27.
4. Penzien DB, Rains JC, Andrasik F, et al. Behavioral management of recurrent headache: three decades of experience and empiricism. Appl Psychophysiol Biofeedback 2002;27:163–81.
5. Coulter ID, Favreau JT, Hardy ML, et al. Biofeedback interventions for gastrointestinal conditions: a systematic review. Altern Ther Health Med 2002;8:76–83.
6. Flor H, Birbaumer N. Comparison of the efficacy of electromyographic biofeedback, cognitive–behavioral therapy, and conservative medical interventions in the treatment of chronic musculoskeletal pain. J Consult Clin Psychol 1993;61: 653–8.
7. Karlstrom E, Abel GG. Biofeedback for musculoskeletal pain. JAMA 1993;270: 2736.
8. Babu AS, Mathew E, Danda D, et al. Management of patients with fibromyalgia using biofeedback: a randomized control trial. Indian J Med Sci 2007;61:455–61.
9. Hassett AL, Radvanski DC, Vaschillo EG, et al. A pilot study of the efficacy of heart rate variability (HRV) biofeedback in patients with fibromyalgia. Appl Psychophysiol Biofeedback 2007;32:1–10.
10. Kayiran S, Dursun E, Ermutlu N, et al. Neurofeedback in fibromyalgia syndrome. Agri 2007;19:47–53.
11. Crider A, Glaros AG, Gevirtz RN, et al. Efficacy of biofeedback-based treatments for temporomandibular disorders. Appl Psychophysiol Biofeedback 2005;30: 333–45.
12. Leins U, Goth G, Hinterberger T, et al. Neurofeedback for children with ADHD: a comparison of SCP and Theta/Beta protocols. Appl Psychophysiol Biofeedback 2007;32:73–88.
13. Toplak ME, Connors L, Shuster J, et al. Review of cognitive, cognitive-behavioral, and neural-based interventions for Attention-Deficit/Hyperactivity Disorder (ADHD). Clin Psychol Rev 2008;28:801–23.
14. Glazer HI, Laine CD, Glazer HI, et al. Pelvic floor muscle biofeedback in the treatment of urinary incontinence: a literature review. Appl Psychophysiol Biofeedback 2006;31:187–201.
15. Sterman MB, Egner T. Foundation and practice of neurofeedback for the treatment of epilepsy. Appl Psychophysiol Biofeedback 2006;31:21–35.

16. Bigger JT, Fleiss JL, Rolnitzky LM, et al. The ability of several short-term measures of RR variability to predict mortality after myocardial infarction. Circulation 1993;88:927–34.

17. Kleiger RE, Miller JP, Bigger JT Jr, et al. Decreased heart rate variability and its association with increased mortality after acute myocardial infarction. Am J Cardiol 1987;59:256–62.

18. Logtenberg SJ, Kleefstra N, Houweling ST, et al. Effect of device-guided breathing exercises on blood pressure in hypertensive patients with type 2 diabetes mellitus: a randomized controlled trial. J Hypertens 2007;25:241–6.

19. Moravec CS, Moravec CS. Biofeedback therapy in cardiovascular disease: rationale and research overview. Cleve Clin J Med 2008;75(Suppl 2):S35–8.

20. Schein MH, Gavish B, Baevsky T, et al. Treating hypertension in type II diabetic patients with device-guided breathing: a randomized controlled trial. J Hum Hypertens 2009;23:325–31.

21. Lehrer P, Smetankin A, Potapova T. Respiratory sinus arrhythmia biofeedback therapy for asthma: a report of 20 unmedicated pediatric cases using the Smetankin method. Appl Psychophysiol Biofeedback 2000;25:193–200.

22. Lehrer P, Vaschillo E, Lu SE, et al. Heart rate variability biofeedback: effects of age on heart rate variability, baroreflex gain, and asthma. Chest 2006;129:278–84.

23. Lehrer PM, Vaschillo E, Vaschillo B, et al. Biofeedback treatment for asthma. Chest 2004;126:352–61.

24. McKay E, Kaufman RH, Doctor U, et al. Treating vulvar vestibulitis with electromyographic biofeedback of pelvic floor musculature. J Reprod Med 2001;46:337–42.

25. Karavidas MK, Tsai PS, Yucha C, et al. Thermal biofeedback for primary Raynaud's phenomenon: a review of the literature. Appl Psychophysiol Biofeedback 2006;31:203–16.

26. Chiarioni G, Heymen S, Whitehead WE, et al. Biofeedback therapy for dyssynergic defecation. World J Gastroenterol 2006;12:7069–74.

27. Heymen S, Jones KR, Scarlett Y, et al. Biofeedback treatment of constipation: a critical review. Dis Colon Rectum 2003;46:1208–17.

28. Norton C, Cody JD, Hosker G. Biofeedback and/or sphincter exercises for the treatment of faecal incontinence in adults [update of Cochrane Database Syst Rev 2000;(2):CD002111; PMID: 10796859]. Cochrane Database Syst Rev 2006;(3):CD002111.

29. Aapb, Bcia, ISNR. Task force to establish definition of biofeedback 2008. Available at: http://www.aapb.org/consumers_biofeedback.html.

30. Schwartz M. Biofeedback: a practitioner's guide. 3rd edition. New York: Guilford Press; 2003.

31. Barnes PM, Bloom B, Nahin RL, et al. Complementary and alternative medicine use among adults and children: United States, 2007. Natl Health Stat Report 2009;1–23.

32. Berntson GG, Bigger JT Jr, Eckberg DL, et al. Heart rate variability: origins, methods, and interpretive caveats. Psychophysiology 1997;34:623–48.

33. Friel PN. EEG biofeedback in the treatment of attention deficit hyperactivity disorder. Altern Med Rev 2007;12:146–51.

34. McCraty R, Atkinson M, Tomasino D, et al. The impact of an emotional self-management skills course on psychosocial functioning and autonomic recovery to stress in middle school children. Integr Physiol Behav Sci 1999;34:246–68.

35. Lehrer PM, Vaschillo E, Vaschillo B. Resonant frequency biofeedback training to increase cardiac variability: rationale and manual for training. Appl Psychophysiol Biofeedback 2000;25:177–91.

Acupuncture in Primary Care

Jun J. Mao, MD, MSCE[a],*, Rahul Kapur, MD, CAQSM[b]

KEYWORDS

- Acupuncture/history/standards
- Acupuncture therapy/adverse effects • China
- Evidence-based medicine • Meta-analysis • Primary care

Acupuncture is a traditional Chinese medical therapy that uses hair-thin metal needles to puncture the skin at specific points on the body to relieve pain and promote well-being. In this article, we provide a historical and philosophic overview of acupuncture and describe its current use in the United States. We then synthesize the basic scientific theory of acupuncture and present recent clinical evidence of how acupuncture may be used for a broad category of diseases, with a specific focus on conditions common to a primary care clinic, including low back pain, osteoarthritis, neck pain, and headache. We also discuss the practical issues concerning the integration of acupuncture into primary care to create coordinated, patient-centered care.

A CASE PRESENTATION

Ms Smith (not her real name) is an 82-year-old woman with a history of hypertension and high cholesterol. She presented with 6 months of low back pain. She denied any acute onset of pain. She described her pain as fairly constant, worse with standing and walking, and relieved by sitting. However, prolonged sitting could make the pain worse as well, she said. She described the pain as achy in nature and sometimes traveled down along her left buttock. On a scale of 0 to 10, with 1 being no pain and 10 being the most intense pain, she rated the pain as 6 out of 10 on average and 10 out of 10 at worst. She lives by herself and said the pain interfered with her sleep and made taking

Dr Mao is supported by National Institutes of Health–National Center for Complementary and Alternative Medicine (NIH/NCCAM) grant 1 K23 AT004112 and an American Cancer Society Cancer Control Career Development Award for Primary Care Physicians. The grant agencies played no role in shaping the content of this manuscript. Dr Mao is the founder and president of Acupuncture Education International, Inc.

[a] Department of Family Medicine and Community Health, University of Pennsylvania, 2 Gates Building, 3400 Spruce Street, Philadelphia, PA 19104, USA
[b] Department of Family Medicine and Community Health, University of Pennsylvania Sports Medicine Center, University of Pennsylvania Health System, 51 North 39th Street, Mutch Building 6th Floor, Philadelphia, PA 19104, USA
* Corresponding author.
E-mail address: maoj@uphs.upenn.edu (J.J. Mao).

Prim Care Clin Office Pract 37 (2010) 105–117
doi:10.1016/j.pop.2009.09.010
primarycare.theclinics.com

care of herself difficult. She has become frustrated by the pain and is anxious and depressed at the thought that she may lose her independence because of the pain. During the past several months, she was evaluated by her primary care physician (PCP), an orthopedic doctor, and a pain specialist. Her lumbar MRI showed mild lumbar stenosis at the L4-L5 region. She has been taking naproxen but has only experienced mild relief. She said the when she takes "too much," her stomach becomes uncomfortable. She had a brief course of physical therapy, which did not seem to help much. She was recommended to have an epidural treatment. However, she is afraid of the "needle going into the back" and would want to try something noninvasive first. Her friends suggested trying acupuncture and she asked her PCP about it. The PCP told her, "It probably won't hurt. Why don't you give it a try?"

When Dr Mao evaluated Ms Smith, she appeared to be younger than her stated age and slightly anxious. She did not really understand acupuncture, nor did she have high expectations for its effectiveness. However, she was willing to give it a try because it has helped her friend. Mrs Smith walked into the office with a cane. Her range of motion of the lumbar area was poor with limited flexion. She had mild kyphosis with no bony tenderness on palpation. It took her a long time to climb onto the examination table and find a comfortable position. Specific trigger points were palpated at 2 cm lateral to the L5 area, around the sacral iliac joint, and in the left gluteal maximus region. Dr Mao performed acupuncture for seven sessions for her. She had minimal improvement during the first two treatments. However, she found the treatments calming and relaxing. When she returned for the fourth treatment, she felt "something definitely has changed." She no longer needs the cane when walking, and the pain is never 10 out of 10 any more. At this point, Dr Mao instructed her to see a physical therapist to strengthen her core muscle and then spaced her visits to every 2 weeks. With an additional three treatments, her pain decreased to 1 or 2 out of 10 and now minimally bothers her. Because acupuncture is not covered by her insurance, she and Dr Mao agreed that she no longer needs to get acupuncture, will continue with physical therapy for strengthening, and will return as needed.

HISTORICAL PERSPECTIVE

Acupuncture is part of the much larger system of healing called traditional Chinese medicine (TCM).[1] TCM is one of the oldest healing systems still used by significant numbers of Chinese and others around the world. In this medical paradigm, therapeutic options include those involving herbs; diet; exercise, such as tai chi; massage (*tuina*); and *qi gong* (energy therapy); in addition to acupuncture. TCM focuses on promoting the "inner balance" or homeostasis of the individual within the larger external environment. Any imbalance is viewed as "illness." One of the many key concepts in TCM is *qi*, a vital energy that circulates throughout the body in 14 channels called meridians. When the flow of *qi* becomes obstructed, pain or illness occurs. Putting needles at specific acupuncture points along the meridian seeks to "open the channel" and promote the healthy flow of *qi* and, with that, restore health.[1,2]

Historians debate about when acupuncture was developed, though some think it originated over 5000 years ago. The earliest source of systematic documentation of acupuncture theory is the *Huang Di Nei Jing* (the *Inner Classic of the Yellow Emperor*), which dates back to the Han dynasty in the second century BC.[2] Like many medical systems, acupuncture theory and practice have evolved over the years in China and in the West. Many similar but different schools emerged, such as the Japanese, Korean, and French energetic styles of acupuncture. With the increasing understanding of neuroscience and anatomy, the practice of acupuncture in China, as well as in the West, has become more neuromuscular-based for some musculoskeletal and neurologic conditions. In the United States, the predominant practice of acupuncture is still TCM based.[3]

WHAT IS ACUPUNCTURE LIKE?

Regardless of the style of acupuncture, the practitioner often uses hair-thin metal needles, which the practitioner inserts in specific acupuncture points along the meridians or at the tender points, known in Chinese medicine as *ashi* points. In the TCM style, the needles are often manipulated until either the physician perceives the needle being grabbed by the tissues or the patient experiences *de qi*, a sensation described as a mixture of heaviness, soreness, distention, tingling, and numbness, which can travel from one place to another.[4] Patients will then lay still for about 20 to 40 minutes. During the acupuncture treatment, the practitioners often perform tongue and pulse diagnosis. Additionally, heat and electric stimulation may be applied to augment the needling sensation. Furthermore, the practitioners, in addition to providing acupuncture treatments, often offer advice on exercise, diet, lifestyle modification, and prescription herbal treatments.[5] In large prospective studies, acupuncture has been found to be very safe, with the most common side effects being needling pain, bruising, hematoma, and dizziness. Very rare cases of severe tiredness, headache, or pneumothorax have been reported for needling the chest area.[6,7] Most patients perceive acupuncture as calming and relaxing.[4] The course of acupuncture treatment typically includes 10 sessions, while many people require fewer and some need more.

CURRENT STATE OF ACUPUNCTURE USE IN THE UNITED STATES

In 2002, approximately 2 million United States adults 18 or older had used acupuncture.[8] By 2007, this number had exceeded 3 million, representing a 50% growth in the 5 years.[9] In the United States, the most common reasons for seeking acupuncture treatment are to relieve low back pain (34%), joint pain (16%), neck pain (14%), and headache/migraine (10%).[10] Among the estimated 2 million users, 44% of individuals sought acupuncture care because conventional medical care would not help, while 57% felt that combining acupuncture with conventional medical care would help. About 25% to 35% of respondents indicated that conventional medical professionals recommended that they seek out acupuncture treatment. Among users, 46% felt acupuncture helped a great deal, 26% had some help, and about 28% perceived that it provided very little or no help.[10]

BASIC SCIENTIFIC BASIS OF ACUPUNCTURE

The exact mechanism of action for acupuncture is not fully understood. Animal and human studies have demonstrated an analgesic effect mediated in part by endogenous opioid release,[11–14] and the non–naloxone-responsive component is blocked by both serotonin and norepinephrine antagonists.[15–18] Recently, neuroimaging techniques, including positron emission tomography scan,[19–21] single-photon emission CT,[22] and functional MRI,[23–26] have provided new ways to study central nervous system acupuncture response. Data suggest that acupuncture may modulate the limbic system,[23,27] which processes the cognitive and emotional aspects of pain in humans. Additionally, the hypothalamus and brainstem networks are also implicated in acupuncture analgesia.[28] Furthermore, it has been suggested that nonspecific effects, such as expectation, may also play an integral part in mediating the central nervous system response to acupuncture.[19,21] Peripherally, animal data suggest that acupuncture may result in local vasodilatation,[29,30] connective tissue displacement and transduction,[31–33] and inhibition of inflammatory response.[34] Based on these basic science findings, the mechanism of acupuncture for chronic pain or other clinical issues is highly complex, recruiting both the central and peripheral networks and eliciting both psychological and physiologic responses in individuals.

CLINICAL EVIDENCE RELATED TO ACUPUNCTURE

Over the last 40 years, thousands of acupuncture clinical trials have been conducted for diverse conditions. Before discussing the clinical evidence, it is important to have an understanding of the challenges of methodology in evaluating acupuncture, particularly the choice of control. The question of what constitutes an appropriate placebo for acupuncture has been debated through the years and remains controversial.[35] Each control helps answer a small and specific question about the effects of acupuncture.[36,37] The needling of sham points—the needling of points other than theorized acupuncture points—has been tried to better understand whether the effect of acupuncture is mediated through specific meridians and points. Shallow/superficial needling has been performed to help determine whether the depth of needling has an effect on the clinical response. The problem with using these control techniques is that skin penetration may excite diffuse noxious inhibitory control,[38] a physiologic response that is not inert. The introduction of Streitberger needles,[39] a needle device that acts like a stage dagger and gives the impression of skin penetration without piercing the skin, helps to delineate whether skin penetration is important in acupuncture therapy. However, such skin tactile stimulation is also not physiologically inert either. Acupuncture research methodologists argue that acupuncture trials ought to be conducted with three arms: true acupuncture, placebo/sham control, and standard medical care. In this way, the specific efficacy of needling effects and clinical relevance of acupuncture as an entire package of care can be evaluated simultaneously.[40]

Clinical Evidence Before 1997

The National Institutes of Health conducted a consensus conference based on review and expert presentation of literature from 1970 to 1997.[41] The conference reached the following conclusions:

> Acupuncture as a therapeutic intervention is widely practiced in the United States. Although there have been many studies of its potential usefulness, many of these studies provide equivocal results because of design, sample size, and other factors. The issue is further complicated by inherent difficulties in the use of appropriate controls, such as placebos and sham acupuncture groups. However, promising results have emerged, for example, showing efficacy of acupuncture in adult postoperative and chemotherapy nausea and vomiting and in postoperative dental pain. There are other situations, such as addiction, stroke rehabilitation, headache, menstrual cramps, tennis elbow, fibromyalgia, myofascial pain, osteoarthritis, low back pain, carpal tunnel syndrome, and asthma, in which acupuncture may be useful as an adjunct treatment or an acceptable alternative or be included in a comprehensive management program. Further research is likely to uncover additional areas where acupuncture interventions will be useful.[41]

This meeting helped lay the foundation for rigorous research in acupuncture over the next decade.

Clinical Evidence After 1997

Since the National Institutes of Health consensus conference, high-quality and well-powered clinical trials have been conducted in the United States and in Europe for low back pain, knee osteoarthritis, neck pain, and headache (**Table 1**). These large clinical trials often show that the effects of acupuncture are clinically relevant, as compared with usual care or enhanced standard care. However, many trials resulted in inconsistent or clinically irrelevant effects of acupuncture when compared with placebo/sham controls. Nevertheless, the effects of acupuncture in these clinical trials often lasted for at least 6 months. Furthermore, acupuncture appeared to reduce the use of medications, improve pain-related quality of life, and reduce time off from work. Several large cost-effectiveness analyses performed in Europe showed that acupuncture is a cost-effective intervention for low back pain,[61] knee osteoarthritis,[62] neck pain,[63] and headache.[56,57]

SPECIFIC CONDITIONS

Musculoskeletal complaints are extremely common in the primary care setting. In 2005, the National Ambulatory Medical Care Survey showed that musculoskeletal problems tied with respiratory complaints as the number one symptom category of patients seeing their family physicians, each with 9.9% of visits.[64] Back pain and knee pain accounted for one third of these visits. In treating these patients, more and more physicians have turned to acupuncture as an adjunct or alternative to conventional treatment. In this section, we hope to provide a summary of the current evidence of the efficacy of acupuncture for both low back pain and knee osteoarthritis.

Acupuncture in Low Back Pain (Grade A Evidence)

As mentioned earlier, back pain is the most common reason for visits to acupuncturists in America.[65] While research in China has overwhelmingly shown that acupuncture is beneficial for treatment of back pain, the research findings throughout the rest of the world have often been inconsistent and controversial.[42] In the past decade, the number of high-quality randomized controlled trials (RCTs) studying acupuncture has increased tremendously. Most of these trials have shown acupuncture to be better than no treatment and at least equivalent to usual care for back pain.[42] A 2005 meta-analysis of acupuncture for low back pain reviewed 22 RCTs and found a small but statistically significant benefit to acupuncture for chronic low back pain (>3 months) when compared with sham acupuncture, sham transcutaneous nerve stimulation, and no additional treatment. Acupuncture was not statistically better than other active

Table 1 Strength of evidence for acupuncture as a treatment for common conditions		
Key Clinical Recommendation on Acupuncture[a]	**Evidence Rating**	**References**
Low back pain: effective	A	42–45
Knee/hip osteoarthritis: effective	A	35,46–50
Headaches: effective	A	51–55
Neck pain: effective	A	56–60

[a] Effectiveness is determined by a comparison between acupuncture and routine care or enhanced medical care. In most studies, the specific effect of acupuncture needling against placebo/sham acupuncture is small and findings are inconsistent.

treatments, such as massage and manipulation. These results were true for both short- and long-term effects (>6-week follow-up).[42]

Since 2005, many European trials have added support for the benefits of acupuncture, but have also stirred up controversy regarding "sham" acupuncture. In 2006, an RCT conducted by Brinkhaus and colleagues[43] found acupuncture to be statistically effective in reducing pain scores when compared to controls receiving no treatment for chronic low back pain (>21-point improvement on 100-point scale at 8 weeks). However, the difference was found to be only 5 points when compared with sham acupuncture and the difference failed to be statistically significant at 26 and 52 weeks. In 2007, the German Acupuncture Trials (GERAC), a randomized, multicenter, blinded parallel-group trial, compared acupuncture, sham acupuncture, and conventional therapy, following patient outcomes for 6 months after treatment. Both acupuncture and sham acupuncture had statistically significant response rates when compared with conventional therapy (47.6% and 44.2% vs 27.4%) at 6 months.[44] More recently, Cherkin and colleagues[45] conducted an RCT comparing acupuncture, noninsertive sham acupuncture, and usual care. They again found a statistically significant difference between acupuncture groups (sham and traditional) and usual care at 8 weeks and 26 weeks.[45]

Acupuncture in Knee Osteoarthritis (Grade A Evidence)

As our patient population ages, the prevalence of patients suffering from knee osteoarthritis will continue to rise. Knee pain already affects 25% of patients over 55,[46] and one study showed that 70% of patients over the age of 50 with knee pain already have radiographic evidence of knee arthritis.[66] Because there is no definitive cure for osteoarthritis, current treatments are aimed at reducing pain and improving function in hopes of delaying knee-replacement surgery. As with back pain, acupuncture is being used with increased frequency as an adjunct or alternative to both pharmacologic and nonpharmacologic treatment of knee osteoarthritis, and is a common reason for referral to acupuncturists.[10] Like the evidence related to back pain, the evidence for acupuncture for knee osteoarthritis is varied, especially in comparison to sham acupuncture.

Much of the research on acupuncture within this decade has been done in Germany. In the Acupuncture Research Trials (ARTs), acupuncture and sham acupuncture were compared with a wait-list control group for four common conditions, including knee osteoarthritis.[35] The primary outcome was determined by pain scores on the Western Ontario and McMaster University Osteoarthritis (WOMAC) index at 8-week follow-up. After 8 weeks, the mean baseline-adjusted WOMAC index was 26.9 in the acupuncture group, 35.8 in the sham acupuncture group, and 49.6 in the control group. Treatment differences were −8.8 for acupuncture versus sham acupuncture and −22.7 for acupuncture versus waiting list, both statistically significant. In the acupuncture group, the success rate (defined as a 50% improvement in WOMAC score) was 52%, as compared with 28% and 3% in the sham acupuncture and control groups, respectively.[47]

In 2006, Witt and colleagues[48] followed the above study with the Acupuncture in Routine Care study, a multicenter RCT with a nonrandomized arm. This study found acupuncture to be an effective adjunct to routine care for both hip and knee osteoarthritis. At 3 months, the acupuncture group had a WOMAC score of 30.5 (change of 17.6) as compared with a score of 47.3 (change of 0.9) in the control group receiving usual care. The success rate was 34.5% in the acupuncture group as compared with 6.5% in the control group.

Alongside the ARTs, the GERAC trials were being conducted to compare acupuncture to sham acupuncture and guideline-oriented standard therapy. Unlike ARTs though, GERAC found very little difference between acupuncture and sham acupuncture. In results published by Scharf and colleagues[49] in 2006, the success rates (defined as a 36% improvement in WOMAC scores at 13 and 26 weeks) were 53.1% for acupuncture, 51.0% for sham acupuncture, and 29.1% for standard therapy. Both acupuncture and sham acupuncture were significantly better than standard therapy. Adding to this data, a 2007 meta-analysis of nine RCTs found acupuncture to be significantly better in short-term pain and function improvement as compared with wait-list control groups, but not significantly better than sham acupuncture.[50] These studies again raise questions as to whether sham acupuncture is truly inert. Another study illustrating this controversy was a systematic review and meta-analysis of only those RCTs that included "true sham" acupuncture, defined as an acupuncturelike procedure that did not stimulate any nerves of the knee joint.[46] The investigators also strictly defined "adequate" acupuncture based on sessions, points needled, length of session, and adequate sensation produced. When studies comparing "adequate" acupuncture to "true sham" acupuncture were analyzed, acupuncture was found to be significantly superior to sham acupuncture for both pain and function WOMAC scores in both the short and long term.[46]

Neck Pain (Grade A Evidence)

A systematic review in 1999 analyzing 14 trials found that acupuncture was effective compared with one wait-list control in 1 trial, either superior to or equal to physiotherapy in 3 studies, and had similar results to sham/placebo control.[51] Since then, acupuncture has been found to be superior to massage[52] and dry needling[53] in treating motion-related neck pain. In a recent trial of acupuncture compared with placebo, acupuncture was found to have statistically significant but clinically irrelevant benefits.[54] In a large pragmatic RCT (1880 randomized to acupuncture, 1886 to routine care only) nested in a large cohort study (N = 14,161), acupuncture was found to have clinically relevant improvement for pain and disability ($P<.001$) at 3 months and improvement persisted for 6 months at the final follow-up. The nonrandomized cohort of acupuncture patients had more severe symptoms at baseline and showed greater improvement than the randomized patients who received acupuncture.[55]

Headache (Grade A Evidence)

In a large epidemiology study conducted in Germany involving patients with migraines, episodic headaches, or chronic tensionlike headaches (N = 2022), 53% of patients reported that headache frequency decreased by 50% or more. Clinical improvement is also seen in other outcomes and in quality of life.[58] A recent systematic review summarizing 11 trials of acupuncture for tensionlike headache with 2317 patients found that acupuncture had statistically significant and clinically relevant benefit over routine care for both headache frequency and pain intensity. Of the 6 trials comparing acupuncture with sham, 5 showed that acupuncture had statistically significant and clinically relevant benefit. Meanwhile the 4 trials comparing acupuncture against massage, physical therapy, or relaxation had significant methodological limitations, as data were difficult to interpret, and showed slightly better outcomes than control interventions.[59] In 2 cost-effectiveness trials, 1 conducted in Germany[56] and 1 in England,[57] acupuncture was found to be cost-effective when implemented into primary care networks for headaches. In a study conducted among headache patients seen in neurology headache specialty clinics, the integration of acupuncture into ongoing medical management offered not only clinically relevant reductions in headache frequency and severity but also improvements in headache-related quality of life.[60]

PUTTING CLINICAL EVIDENCE INTO PATIENT-CENTERED CARE

In analyzing these trials as a whole, the consistent take-home message is that acupuncture is effective for the treatment of chronic painful symptoms when compared with no treatment, routine care, or even enhanced care of short-term efficacy. The achieved effects of acupuncture appear to last over a long-term period (6 months). Therefore, acupuncture seems to be a reasonable adjunct or alternative to offer to patients for whom usual care is ineffective or unsatisfactory. What is less clear is why sham acupuncture also produces similar improvements. A recent study by Harris and colleagues[67] using C-carfentanil positron emission tomography imaging, found that, while both real and sham acupuncture produced similar clinical benefit for patients with fibromyalgia, the mechanism underlying the pain reduction is different. Real acupuncture increased both short- and long-term mu-opioid receptor binding potential in multiple pain and sensory processing regions, while sham acupuncture actually resulted in only a small reduction. This study suggests that the pathways that acupuncture and sham acupuncture use to produce clinical effects may be different.

EDUCATION OF PHYSICIANS IN ACUPUNCTURE

While an estimated 16,000 nonphysician acupuncturists practice in the United States, 6000 physicians have the training to incorporate acupuncture into their practices.[10] PCPs continue to dominate the physician-acupuncturist population, although anesthesiologists and pain management specialists make up significant proportions.[68] Ten acupuncture training programs are certified by the American Board of Medical Acupuncture for doctors. Each program requires at least 300 hours of training, 100 of which involves acupuncture-specific training. These programs vary not only in format, from video-based learning to conventional in-person courses, but also vary in their systems of acupuncture training.[69] Some information can be found on line on acupuncture and acupuncture training (**Box 1**).

PRACTICAL CONCERNS FOR INTEGRATING ACUPUNCTURE INTO PRIMARY CARE

There are two ways to integrate acupuncture into primary care and thus provide patients with more therapeutic options. One is to establish a trusted and competent referral partner who practices acupuncture. With close collaboration, the acupuncturist can address patients' clinical issues while the PCP coordinates care. Another way is to obtain additional training through the above-discussed certified courses. This is particularly useful for those PCPs who like a hands-on approach to patients.

Box 1
Useful acupuncture Internet resources

Acupuncture information for patients: National Center for Complementary and Alternative Medicine (http://nccam.nih.gov/health/acupuncture/)

Acupuncture training programs for physicians: American Academy of Medical Acupuncture (http://www.dabma.org/programs.asp)

Overseas acupuncture program for medical students: Acupuncture Education International

To be a good acupuncturist requires not only the skills but also the right temperament because most patients seen have with chronic pain and have been treated by conventional approaches, which have failed, or favor a nontraditional view of medicine or health. A clinician needs more than skills to build a successful acupuncture practice. He or she also must be able to establish an empathic and nurturing relationship with patients and to remain open-minded. Acupuncture skills can be further honed with continued medical education in acupuncture and self-directed learning. As one transitions into a physician acupuncturist, the role of a PCP may shift into that of a specialist. In that case, the clinician may find it helpful to establish a network of physician or health care provider partners to serve as a referral base. Some specific examples of such partners include other PCPs, sports medicine physicians, physical medicine and rehabilitation physicians, oncologists, and physical therapists. In building an acupuncture practice, the clinician will face barriers, such as time limitations and financial constraints.[68] However, with determination, a combination of skills, and compassion, the practice of acupuncture in the context of primary care can be very rewarding both financially and psychologically as it help creates a holistic healing environment.

PATIENT-PHYSICIAN COMMUNICATION IN REGARDS TO ACUPUNCTURE CARE

The essence of evidence-based medicine rests on the shared decision making with patients by aligning patients' preference with the best available evidence for the specific health conditions in the context of patients' social, cultural, and financial circumstances. The discussion of acupuncture in the context of conventional medicine not only needs to cover the efficacy of acupuncture and various therapies, but also their safety and potential harm. Secondly, because acupuncture is not covered by insurance in many states, patients with financial concerns should instead be offered therapy options covered by insurance, such as physical therapy or chiropractic care, as long as the patient has no particular preference. Third, with acupuncture as with any therapy, some people respond and some do not. Therefore, realistic expectations need to be set for patients. We often require patients to have at least a verbal commitment of six treatments before starting treatment. Although many patients may not need even six treatments to experience benefits, a commitment on the part of the patient may help reduce the likelihood of disappointing outcomes stemming from insufficient treatment. Lastly, many patients who seek acupuncture may be using multiple conventional and complementary therapies. We often ask them to avoid using two therapies (eg, acupuncture and massage) within a 24-hour period so that each therapy is allowed to manifest its own effect. More importantly, should an adverse event occurs, the task of determining a cause is easier if just one treatment at a time is used. As a PCP acupuncturist, the time spent with patients during acupuncture treatments also helps to reinforce active coping, self-efficacy, and healthy lifestyle modification, all of which can have additional benefits for patients' overall health beyond the primary reason for seeking care.

SUMMARY

Acupuncture is a safe, traditional Chinese medical therapy that patients often find both calming and relaxing. Animal and human studies have found a physiologic basis for acupuncture needling that involves both central and peripheral networks. Although it is unclear whether real acupuncture is more beneficial than sham/placebo acupuncture, acupuncture care yields both clinically relevant short- and long-term benefits for low back pain, knee osteoarthritis, chronic neck pain, and headache. Also, the integration of acupuncture into a primary care setting appears to be cost-effective for such conditions. The successful practice of acupuncture in primary care requires rigorous training, financial discipline, and good communication skills. When it is done correctly, acupuncture proves to be beneficial for both patients and providers.

ACKNOWLEDGMENTS

We thank Dingyun Chan for performing literature search and technical assistance.

REFERENCES

1. Cheng X, editor. Chinese acupuncture and moxibustion. Beijing (China): Foreign Languages Press; 1987.
2. Kaptchuk TJ. Acupuncture: theory, efficacy, and practice. Ann Intern Med 2002; 136(5):374–83.
3. Sherman KJ, Cherkin DC, Eisenberg DM, et al. The practice of acupuncture: who are the providers and what do they do? Ann Fam Med 2005;3(2):151–8.
4. Mao JJ, Farrar JT, Armstrong K, et al. De qi: Chinese acupuncture patients' experiences and beliefs regarding acupuncture needling sensation—an exploratory survey. Acupunct Med 2007;25(4):158–65.
5. Sherman KJ, Cherkin DC, Deyo RA, et al. The diagnosis and treatment of chronic back pain by acupuncturists, chiropractors, and massage therapists. Clin J Pain 2006;22(3):227–34.
6. Macpherson H, Scullion A, Thomas KJ, et al. Patient reports of adverse events associated with acupuncture treatment: a prospective national survey. Qual Saf Health Care 2004;13(5):349–55.
7. White A. A cumulative review of the range and incidence of significant adverse events associated with acupuncture. Acupunct Med 2004;22(3):122–33.
8. Barnes PM, Powell-Griner E, McFann K, et al. Complementary and alternative medicine use among adults: United States. Adv Data 2002;2004(343):1–19.
9. Barnes PM, Bloom B, Nahin RL. Complementary and alternative medicine use among adults and children: United States, 2007. Natl Health Stat Report 2009(12):1–23.
10. Burke A, Upchurch DM, Dye C, et al. Acupuncture use in the United States: findings from the National Health Interview Survey. J Altern Complement Med 2006; 12(7):639–48.
11. Ulett GA, Han S, Han JS. Electroacupuncture: mechanisms and clinical application. Biol Psychiatry 1998;44(2):129–38.
12. Wu DZ. Acupuncture and neurophysiology. Clin Neurol Neurosurg 1990;92(1): 13–25.
13. Han JS. Acupuncture and endorphins. Neurosci Lett 2003;361(1–3):258–61.
14. Han JS. Acupuncture: neuropeptide release produced by electrical stimulation of different frequencies. Trends Neurosci 2003;26(1):17–22.
15. Xuan YT, Zhou ZF, Wu WY, et al. Anatagonism of acupuncture analgesia and morphine analgesia by cinanserin injected into the nucleus accumbens and habenula in the rabbit. J Beijing Med Coll 1982;14:23–6 [in Chinese].
16. Xu DY, Zhou ZF, Han JS. Amgdaloid serotonin and endogenous opoid substances (OLS) are important for mediating electroacupuncture analgesia and morphine analgesia in rabbit. Acta Physiol Sin 1985;38:19–25 [in Chinese, English abs.]
17. Cheng R, Pomeranz B. Monoamineergic mechanisms of electroacupuncture analgesia. Brain Res 1981;215:77–92.

18. Han JS, Terenius L. Neurochemical basis of acupuncture analgesia. Annu Rev Pharmacol Toxicol 1982;22:193–220.
19. Lewith GT, White PJ, Pariente J. Investigating acupuncture using brain imaging techniques: the current state of play. Evid Based Complement Alternat Med 2005;2(3):315–9.
20. Biella G, Sotgiu ML, Pellegata G, et al. Acupuncture produces central activations in pain regions. Neuroimage 2001;14(1 Pt 1):60–6.
21. Pariente J, White P, Frackowiak RS, et al. Expectancy and belief modulate the neuronal substrates of pain treated by acupuncture. Neuroimage 2005;25(4):1161–7.
22. Newberg AB, Lariccia PJ, Lee BY, et al. Cerebral blood flow effects of pain and acupuncture: a preliminary single-photon emission computed tomography imaging study. J Neuroimaging 2005;15(1):43–9.
23. Hui KK, Liu J, Makris N, et al. Acupuncture modulates the limbic system and subcortical gray structures of the human brain: evidence from fMRI studies in normal subjects. Hum Brain Mapp 2000;9(1):13–25.
24. Fang JL, Krings T, Weidemann J, et al. Functional MRI in healthy subjects during acupuncture: different effects of needle rotation in real and false acupoints. Neuroradiology 2004;46(5):359–62.
25. Napadow V, Makris N, Liu J, et al. Effects of electroacupuncture versus manual acupuncture on the human brain as measured by fMRI. Hum Brain Mapp 2005;24(3):193–205.
26. Wu MT, Sheen JM, Chuang KH, et al. Neuronal specificity of acupuncture response: a fMRI study with electroacupuncture. Neuroimage 2002;16(4):1028–37.
27. Hui KK, Liu J, Marina O, et al. The integrated response of the human cerebro-cerebellar and limbic systems to acupuncture stimulation at ST 36 as evidenced by fMRI. Neuroimage 2005;27(3):479–96.
28. Napadow V, Ahn A, Longhurst J, et al. The status and future of acupuncture mechanism research. J Altern Complement Med 2008;14(7):861–9.
29. Boutouyrie P, Corvisier R, Azizi M, et al. Effects of acupuncture on radial artery hemodynamics: controlled trials in sensitized and naive subjects. Am J Physiol Heart Circ Physiol 2001;280(2):H628–33.
30. Litscher G, Wang L, Huber E, et al. Changed skin blood perfusion in the fingertip following acupuncture needle introduction as evaluated by laser Doppler perfusion imaging. Lasers Med Sci 2002;17(1):19–25.
31. Langevin HM, Yandow JA. Relationship of acupuncture points and meridians to connective tissue planes. Anat Rec 2002;269(6):257–65.
32. Langevin HM, Churchill DL, Wu J, et al. Evidence of connective tissue involvement in acupuncture. FASEB J 2002;16(8):872–4.
33. Langevin HM, Konofagou EE, Badger GJ, et al. Tissue displacements during acupuncture using ultrasound elastography techniques. Ultrasound Med Biol 2004;30(9):1173–83.
34. Chae Y, Hong MS, Kim GH, et al. Protein array analysis of cytokine levels on the action of acupuncture in carrageenan-induced inflammation. Neurol Res 2007;29(Suppl 1):S55–8.
35. Park J, Linde K, Manheimer E, et al. The status and future of acupuncture clinical research. J Altern Complement Med 2008;14(7):871–81.
36. White AR. Acupuncture research methodology. In: Lewith G, Jonas WB, Walach H, editors, Clinical research in complementary therapies: principles, problems and solutions, vol. 1. Edinburgh (United Kingdom): Churchill Livingstone; 2002. p. 307–23.

37. Vickers AJ. Placebo controls in randomized trials of acupuncture. Eval Health Prof 2002;25(4):421–35.
38. Bing Z, Villanueva L, Le Bars D. Acupuncture and diffuse noxious inhibitory controls: naloxone-reversible depression of activities of trigeminal convergent neurons. Neuroscience 1990;37(3):809–18.
39. Streitberger K, Kleinhenz J. Introducing a placebo needle into acupuncture research. Lancet 1998;352(9125):364–5.
40. Langevin HM, Hammerschlag R, Lao L, et al. Controversies in acupuncture research: selection of controls and outcome measures in acupuncture clinical trials. J Altern Complement Med 2006;12(10):943–53.
41. NIH Consensus Conference. Acupuncture. JAMA 1998;280(17):1518–24.
42. Manheimer E, White A, Berman B, et al. Meta-analysis: acupuncture for low back pain. Ann Intern Med 2005;142(8):651–63.
43. Brinkhaus B, Witt CM, Jena S, et al. Acupuncture in patients with chronic low back pain: a randomized controlled trial. Arch Intern Med 2006; 166(4):450–7.
44. Haake M, Muller HH, Schade-Brittinger C, et al. German acupuncture trials (GERAC) for chronic low back pain: randomized, multicenter, blinded, parallel-group trial with 3 groups. Arch Intern Med 2007;167(17):1892–8.
45. Cherkin DC, Sherman KJ, Avins AL, et al. A randomized trial comparing acupuncture, simulated acupuncture, and usual care for chronic low back pain. Arch Intern Med 2009;169(9):858–66.
46. White A, Foster NE, Cummings M, et al. Acupuncture treatment for chronic knee pain: a systematic review. Rheumatology (Oxford) 2007;46(3):384–90.
47. Witt C, Brinkhaus B, Jena S, et al. Acupuncture in patients with osteoarthritis of the knee: a randomised trial. Lancet 2005;366(9480):136–43.
48. Witt CM, Jena S, Brinkhaus B, et al. Acupuncture in patients with osteoarthritis of the knee or hip: a randomized, controlled trial with an additional nonrandomized arm. Arthritis Rheum 2006;54(11):3485–93.
49. Scharf HP, Mansmann U, Streitberger K, et al. Acupuncture and knee osteoarthritis: a three-armed randomized trial. Ann Intern Med 2006;145(1):12–20.
50. Manheimer E, Linde K, Lao L, et al. Meta-analysis: acupuncture for osteoarthritis of the knee. Ann Intern Med 2007;146(12):868–77.
51. White AR, Ernst E. A systematic review of randomized controlled trials of acupuncture for neck pain. Rheumatology (Oxford) 1999;38(2):143–7.
52. Irnich D, Behrens N, Molzen H, et al. Randomised trial of acupuncture compared with conventional massage and "sham" laser acupuncture for treatment of chronic neck pain. BMJ 2001;322(7302):1574–8.
53. Irnich D, Behrens N, Gleditsch JM, et al. Immediate effects of dry needling and acupuncture at distant points in chronic neck pain: results of a randomized, double-blind, sham-controlled crossover trial. Pain 2002;99(1–2):83–9.
54. White P, Lewith G, Prescott P, et al. Acupuncture versus placebo for the treatment of chronic mechanical neck pain: a randomized, controlled trial. Ann Intern Med 2004;141(12):911–9.
55. Witt CM, Jena S, Brinkhaus B, et al. Acupuncture for patients with chronic neck pain. Pain 2006;125(1–2):98–106.
56. Witt CM, Reinhold T, Jena S, et al. Cost-effectiveness of acupuncture treatment in patients with headache. Cephalalgia 2008;28(4):334–45.
57. Vickers AJ, Rees RW, Zollman CE, et al. Acupuncture of chronic headache disorders in primary care: randomised controlled trial and economic analysis. Health Technol Assess 2004;8(48):1–35, iii.

58. Melchart D, Weidenhammer W, Streng A, et al. Acupuncture for chronic head-aches—an epidemiological study. Headache 2006;46(4):632–41.
59. Linde K, Allais G, Brinkhaus B, et al. Acupuncture for tension-type headache. Cochrane Database Syst Rev 2009;(1):CD007587.
60. Coeytaux RR, Kaufman JS, Kaptchuk TJ, et al. A randomized, controlled trial of acupuncture for chronic daily headache. Headache 2005;45(9):1113–23.
61. Ratcliffe J, Thomas KJ, MacPherson H, et al. A randomised controlled trial of acupuncture care for persistent low back pain: cost effectiveness analysis. BMJ 2006;333(7569):626.
62. Reinhold T, Witt CM, Jena S, et al. Quality of life and cost-effectiveness of acupuncture treatment in patients with osteoarthritis pain. Eur J Health Econ 2008;9(3):209–19.
63. Willich SN, Reinhold T, Selim D, et al. Cost-effectiveness of acupuncture treat-ment in patients with chronic neck pain. Pain 2006;125(1–2):107–13.
64. Cherry DK, Woodwell DA, Rechtsteiner EA. National Ambulatory Medical Care Survey: 2005 summary. Adv Data 2007;387:1–39.
65. Cherkin DC, Deyo RA, Sherman KJ, et al. Characteristics of visits to licensed acupuncturists, chiropractors, massage therapists, and naturopathic physicians. J Am Board Fam Pract 2002;15(6):463–72.
66. Duncan RC, Hay EM, Saklatvala J, et al. Prevalence of radiographic osteoar-thritis—it all depends on your point of view. Rheumatology (Oxford) 2006;45(6): 757–60.
67. Harris RE, Zubieta JK, Scott DJ. Traditional Chinese acupuncture and placebo (sham) acupuncture are differentiated by their effects on μ-opioid receptors (MORs). Neuroimage 2009;47(3):1077–85.
68. Yeh GY, Ryan MA, Phillips RS, et al. Doctor training and practice of acupuncture: results of a survey. J Eval Clin Pract 2008;14(3):439–45.
69. American Board of Medical Acupuncture. ABMA approved training programs. URL. Available at: http://www.dabma.org/programs.asp. Accessed June 25, 2009.

Naturopathy and the Primary Care Practice

Sara A. Fleming, ND*, Nancy C. Gutknecht, ND

KEYWORDS

• Naturopathy • Nutrition • Botanical medicine • Homeopathy

NATUROPATHIC MEDICINE OVERVIEW

Naturopathy is a distinct type of primary care medicine that blends age-old healing traditions with scientific advances and current research. Naturopathy is guided by a unique set of principles that recognize the body's innate healing capacity, emphasize disease prevention, and encourage individual responsibility to obtain optimal health (**Box 1**). The naturopathic physician (ND) strives to thoroughly understand each patient's condition, and views symptoms as the body's means of communicating an underlying imbalance. Treatments address the patient's underlying condition, rather than individual presenting symptoms. Modalities used by NDs include diet and clinical nutrition, behavioral change, hydrotherapy, homeopathy, botanical medicine, physical medicine, pharmaceuticals, and minor surgery.[1,2] Naturopathy can be traced back to the European "nature cure," practiced in the nineteenth century, which was a system for treating disease with natural modalities such as water, fresh air, diet, and herbs. In the early twentieth century, naturopathy developed in the United States and Canada, combining nature cure, homeopathy, spinal manipulation, and other therapies (**Fig. 1**).[3]

NATUROPATHIC APPROACH TO HEALTH

In naturopathic theory, illness is viewed as a process of disturbance to health and subsequent recovery in the context of natural systems. Many things can disturb optimal health, such as poor nutrition, chronic stress, or toxic exposure. The goal of the ND is to restore health by identifying and minimizing these disturbances. To do this, the ND first recognizes the factors that determine health (**Table 1**). A determinant becomes a disturbance when it is compromised in some way.

In attempting to restore health, the ND follows a specific, yet adaptable, therapeutic order that begins with minimal interventions and proceeds to higher level interventions as necessary (**Box 2**). The order begins with reestablishing the conditions of health,

Department of Family Medicine, University of Wisconsin-Madison, 1100 Delaplaine Court Madison, WI 53715-1896, USA
* Corresponding author.
E-mail address: sara.fleming@fammed.wisc.edu (S.A. Fleming).

Prim Care Clin Office Pract 37 (2010) 119–136
doi:10.1016/j.pop.2009.09.002
0095-4543/10/$ – see front matter. Published by Elsevier Inc.

primarycare.theclinics.com

Box 1
Principles of naturopathic medicine

- The Healing Power of Nature (Vis Medicatrix Naturae)—Naturopathic medicine recognizes the body's natural healing ability, and trusts that the body has the innate wisdom and intelligence to heal itself if given the proper guidance and tools.
- Identify and Treat the Causes (Tolle Causam)—NDs attempt to identify and treat the underlying cause of illness, rather than focusing on individual presenting symptoms.
- First Do No Harm (Primum Non Nocere)—NDs begin with minimal interventions and proceed to higher level interventions only as determined necessary.
- Doctor as Teacher (Docere)—NDs educate patients, involve them in the healing process, and emphasize the importance of the doctor-patient relationship.
- Treat the Whole Person—Naturopathic medicine takes into account all aspects of an individual's health including physical, mental, emotional, genetic, environmental, social, and spiritual factors.
- Prevention—Naturopathic medicine emphasizes optimal wellness and the prevention of disease.

---

such as developing a more healthful dietary and lifestyle regime. Next, the body's natural healing mechanisms may be stimulated through techniques such as hydrotherapy, which can increase the circulation of blood and lymph. The third step is to support weakened or damaged systems with homeopathy, botanical medicine, or specific exercises, such as yoga. The fourth step is to correct structural integrity, which is typically done with physical medicine techniques including massage and naturopathic manipulation. The fifth step is to address pathology using specific natural substances, such as dietary supplements. The sixth step is to address pathology using pharmaceutical or synthetic substances. Surgical correction is reserved for the final therapeutic step.[4]

CURRENT PRACTICE
Education

NDs are trained over 4 years at accredited doctoral-level naturopathic medical schools. Such schools have been experiencing significant increases in enrollment and graduating class sizes over the past 20 years, particularly since the year 2000.[5] There are currently 7 naturopathic medical schools in the United States and Canada that are either accredited or are in candidate status for accreditation (**Table 2**). The range of didactic instruction at these schools is between 2580 and 3270 hours, and clinical instruction is between 1200 and 1500 hours.[1,6]

Accredited naturopathic medical schools must attain both regional and programmatic accreditation. Regional accreditation is through one of the US Department of Education–recognized regional associations of schools and colleges. Programmatic accreditation for all naturopathic medical schools in North America is through the Council on Naturopathic Medical Education (CNME). All accredited naturopathic medical schools are supported by the Association of Accredited Naturopathic Medical Colleges (AANMC), which acts to promote the naturopathic profession by ensuring rigorous educational standards.[7,8]

Candidates for admission to naturopathic medical school are required to hold a baccalaureate degree, and to have completed all standard premedical undergraduate course work prior to matriculation. The first 2 years of naturopathic medical education

Vincent Priessnitz
1798-1852

Founder of "nature cure," and well-known for his hydrotherapeutic institution in Grafenberg, Germany.

Sebastian Kneipp
1824-1897

Known worldwide for his successful nature cure techniques, which integrated hydrotherapeutic treatments with herbs.

Ernst Schweninger
1850-1924

Established the first nature cure hospital in Grosslichterfelde, Germany.

Heinrich Lahmann
1860-1905

The first nature doctor who graduated from medical schoo.l. Dr. Lahmann founded a hydrotherapy sanatorium, which incorporated raw vegetarian diets.

Henry Lindlahr
1862-1924

Naturopath who established a successful sanitarium for nature cure and osteopathy in Chicago, Illinois. Among other scientific contributions, Dr. Lindlahr wrote Nature Cure, which at its time was considered "the best work ever published in Nature Cure Literature."

Franz Schonenberger
1865-1933

The first university professor who introduced nature cure methods into the Priessneiz Hospital in Berlin, Germany.

Louisa Lust
1868-1925

Known as the "Matriarch of Naturopathy," as she was a successful naturopath specializing in the treatment of women.

Benedict Lust
1872-1945

Known as the "Father of Naturopathy" for his combination of nature cure with homeopathy, massage, spinal manipulation and therapeutic electricity.

Otis G. Carroll
1879-1962

Dr. of chiropractic medicine who invented constitutional hydrotherapy and developed the first means for discerning food sensitivities.

Alfred Brauchle
1898-1964

Conducted "The Great Nature Cure Experiment" in the Johannstadter Hospital in Dresden, Germany. This was the first collaboration between natural and orthodox medical providers.

John Bastyr
1912-1995

Dr. of chiropractic and naturopathic medicine who is known as the "Father of Modern Naturopathic Medicine." Dr. Bastyr founded Bastyr University, located in Seattle, WA.

Fig. 1. Timeline of pioneers in naturopathic medicine. (*Data from* Kirchfeld F, Boyle W. Eclectic therapies. In: Nature doctors: pioneers in naturopathic medicine. Portland, Oregon: Medicina Biologica; 1994.)

focuses on basic and diagnostic sciences including anatomy, physiology, biochemistry, histology, pathology, embryology, neuroscience, immunology, pharmacology, physical and clinical diagnosis, and laboratory diagnosis. The final 2 years of naturopathic medical education focuses on clinical sciences and practicum. Course work specific to naturopathic medicine is woven throughout the program, which includes naturopathic theory, diet and nutrient therapy, botanical medicine, homeopathy, hydrotherapy, massage, naturopathic manipulation, therapeutic exercise, counseling, and case management. Some NDs receive additional training in related disciplines, such as midwifery, Oriental herbal medicine, or acupuncture.[1,7] NDs may choose to specialize in certain populations, such as pediatrics, or certain modalities, such as homeopathy.

Table 1 Determinants of health	
Inborn	Genetic makeup (genotype)
	Intrauterine/congenital
	Maternal exposures
	-Drugs
	-Toxins
	-Viruses
	-Psychoemotional
	Maternal nutrition
	Maternal lifestyle
	Constitution—determines susceptibility
Hygienic factors/lifestyle factors—how we live	Environment, lifestyle, psychoemotional, and spiritual health
	-Spiritual life
	-Self-assessment
	-Relationship to larger universe
	Exposure to Nature
	-Fresh air
	-Clean water
	-Light
	Diet, nutrition, and digestion
	-Unadulterated food
	-Toxemia
	Rest and exercise
	-Rest
	-Exercise
	Socioeconomic factors
	-Culture
	-Loving and being loved
	-Meaningful work
	-Community
	Stress (physical, emotional)
	-Trauma (physical/emotional)
	-Illnesses: pathobiography
	-Medical interventions (or lack of)
	-Surgeries
	-Suppressions
	-Physical and emotional exposures, stresses, and trauma
	-Toxic and harmful substances
	-Addictions

From Zeff J, Snider P, Pizzorno JE. Section I: Philosophy of natural medicine. The textbook of natural medicine, 3rd edition 2006;1(1); with permission.

There are a limited number of 1- to 2-year postdoctoral CNME-certified naturopathic residency programs available. At present, residency is not required for licensure except in Utah. Programs are extremely competitive, with an average of 350 to 400 new ND graduates in the United States per year, and only 30 to 40 openings. Most of these programs are offered through accredited naturopathic medical schools and affiliated clinics, although other opportunities are emerging. An Integrative Medicine Residency is available through several hospitals and clinics, which gives NDs the opportunity to collaborate with conventional medical practitioners. The naturopathic profession has a commitment to increase clinical training opportunities, including the availability of postdoctoral residencies. There is a common informal practice of mentorship in which a new graduate joins the practice of a senior ND.[9]

> **Box 2**
> **Naturopathic therapeutic order**
>
> 1. Establish the conditions for health
>   - Identify and remove disturbing factors
>   - Institute a more healthful regimen
> 2. Stimulate the healing power of nature (vis medicatrix naturae): the self-healing processes
> 3. Address weakened or damaged systems or organs
>   - Strengthen the immune system
>   - Decrease toxicity
>   - Normalize inflammatory function
>   - Optimize metabolic function
>   - Balance regulatory systems
>   - Enhance regeneration
>   - Harmonize life force
> 4. Correct structural integrity
> 5. Address pathology: use specific natural substances, modalities, or interventions
> 6. Address pathology: use specific pharmacologic or synthetic substances
> 7. Suppress or surgically remove pathology
>
> *From* Zeff J, Snider P, Pizzorno JE. Section I: philosophy of natural medicine. The textbook of natural medicine, 3rd edition 2006;1(1); with permission.

Licensing

The licensing of NDs is determined at the state or province level in countries that regulate the profession. At present, Alaska, Arizona, British Columbia, California, Connecticut, the District of Columbia, Hawaii, Idaho, Kansas, Maine, Manitoba, Minnesota, Montana, New Hampshire, Ontario, Oregon, Saskatchewan, Utah, Vermont, and Washington, the United States territories of Puerto Rico and the US Virgin Islands, as well as provinces in Australia and New Zealand, have licensing laws for NDs.[2] Licensing efforts for NDs are led by state organizations, and many currently unlicensed states are in various stages of the process toward licensure. Proximity to an already licensed state is a significant predictor of new licensure.[10] To be eligible for licensure, an ND must have graduated from an accredited naturopathic medical school, and have passed the Naturopathic Physicians Licensing Examination (NPLEx). NPLEx follows the same standards as the National Board of Medical Examiners (for the USMLE), the National Board of Chiropractic Examiners, the National Board of Osteopathic Medical Examiners, and other health care professions.[11]

Licensing laws for NDs increase public safety by ensuring consistency of education, professional standards, compliance with public health standards, appropriate regulation, and currency of continuing education. In states and territories that do not have ND licensing laws, there has been an emergence of unqualified practitioners who did not graduate from appropriately accredited naturopathic medical schools.

Table 2
Accredited naturopathic medical schools in the United States and Canada

School	Contact
Bastyr University	14500 Juanita Drive NE Kenmore, WA 98028 http://www.bastyr.edu/
Boucher Institute of Naturopathic Medicine	300–435 Columbia Street New Westminster, BC V3L 5N8, Canada http://www.binm.org/
Canadian College of Naturopathic Medicine	1255 Sheppard Avenue East Toronto, ON M2K 1E2, Canada http://www.ccnm.edu/
National College of Natural Medicine	049 SW Porter Street Portland, OR 97201 http://www.ncnm.edu/
National University of Health Sciences	200 E. Roosevelt Road Lombard, IL 60148 http://www.nuhs.edu/
Southwest College of Naturopathic Medicine	2140 E. Broadway Road Tempe, AZ 85282 http://www.scnm.edu/
University of Bridgeport	126 Park Avenue Bridgeport, CT 06604 https://www.bridgeport.edu/

Licensure in all areas will protect patients by ensuring that the providers they choose have an education in safe practice of naturopathic medicine.[7]

Scope of Practice

NDs are trained as primary care physicians with an emphasis in natural medicine in ambulatory settings. Their scope of practice varies by state and territory, but generally consists of the diagnosis, prevention, and treatment of disease by stimulation and support of the body's natural healing mechanisms. Standard diagnostic and preventive techniques used include physical examination, laboratory testing, and diagnostic imaging. NDs may employ additional laboratory tests and examination procedures for further evaluation of nutritional status, metabolic functioning, and toxicities. Treatment modalities used by NDs include diet and clinical nutrition, behavioral change, hydrotherapy, homeopathy, botanical medicine, and physical medicine. Depending on the state, NDs may also be licensed to perform minor office procedures and surgery, administer vaccinations, and prescribe many prescriptive drugs.[12]

Insurance Credentialing

An increasing number of insurance companies, unions, and state organizations are credentialing licensed NDs. NDs are not credentialed in the same manner as are medical doctors (MDs) and osteopaths (DOs), because the scope of practice of NDs is not uniform nationwide. The process is based on each state's individual licensing laws and particulars of each company.[7,12] Excessive standardization to cater to credentialing needs may be unfavorable to both NDs and their patients, as individualized care is fundamental to the profession. If the widespread credentialing of NDs is undertaken, a balance between establishing tight practice regulations and allowing for individualized approaches may be necessary.[13]

NDs have been licensed in Washington State since 1919, and credentialed since 1996. An epidemiologic study found that 1.6% of 600,000 enrollees from 3 major insurance companies in Washington filed claims for naturopathic services in 2002,[14] compared with National Health Statistics Reports (NHSR) population-based use estimates of 0.2% for naturopathic services in 2002 and 0.3% in 2007. The increase in use from 2002 to 2007 was, in part, attributed to the increase in naturopathic licensure during that time.[15] Although not a direct comparison, these findings suggest that licensing and credentialing NDs, as in Washington, increases the usage of naturopathic services.

Naturopathic Profession

At the beginning of 2006, there were 4010 licensed NDs in the United States and Canada. This figure represents a 91% increase from 2001.[16] Distance from naturopathic school and population density account for more than 69% of the distribution of NDs, the same factors that predict the distribution of MDs.[17] NDs typically work in private practice, but are also employed by hospitals, clinics, community health centers, universities, and private industry.[1,2] For NDs in private practice in Washington State, an estimated 78.9% reported sharing their office with other providers. These sharers included other NDs (65.2%), acupuncturists (40.4%), massage therapists (40.4%), chiropractors (18.0%), MDs (13.7%), PhDs (6.8%), counselors (6.2%), registered nurses (5.0%), midwives (4.4%), and nutritionists (4.4%).[18]

Within the licensed states of Washington and Connecticut, 75% of all visits to NDs were for chronic conditions, 20% were for acute conditions, and 5% were for wellness/preventive purposes. The most common complaints of patients seeking naturopathic care were fatigue, headache, musculoskeletal problems, anxiety/depression, menopausal symptoms, bowel and abdominal problems, allergies, and rash. The most common pediatric visits in Washington were for health supervision (27.4% of visits), infection (20.6% of visits), and mental health conditions (12.7% of visits). The majority of patients seen were middle-aged Caucasian women. Children were seen in 10.2% to 12.8% of visits, and individuals older than 65 years were seen in 7.8% to 9.7% of visits.[19–21]

More than 70% of ND visits in Washington and Connecticut included physical examination or ordering laboratory/diagnostic tests. The most common examinations were vitals (28%–39% of visits), HEENT (15%–18% of visits), and complete physical (9%–13% of visits). The most frequent laboratory tests were complete blood panels and serum chemistries, which were ordered in 7% to 10% of visits. Other laboratory tests were ordered less frequently and included thyroid panels, lipid panels, allergy tests, stool analyses, urine analyses, vitamin/mineral tests, endocrine, allergy skin tests, and tuberculosis skin tests. Diagnostic imaging, including radiography and ultrasound, was ordered in 1% to 2% of visits. The most common treatments used were botanical medicine (43%–51% of visits), vitamins (41%–43% of visits), minerals (35%–39% of visits), therapeutic diet (26%–36% of visits), homeopathy (19%–29% of visits), and self-care education (17%–23% of visits). Modalities used less frequently included allergy treatment, acupuncture, glandular therapies, manipulation, exercise therapy, hydrotherapy, physiotherapy, mechanotherapy, ultrasound, and mental health counseling. Four percent of all visits included a referral to an MD, and 1% to 2% included a referral to another type of practitioner. The average visit lasted 40 minutes.[19] In pediatric visits in Washington, NDs administered immunizations during 18.6% of health supervision visits for children younger than 2 years, and during 27.3% of visits for children aged from 2 to 5 years.[18]

NATUROPATHIC MODALITIES
Diet and Clinical Nutrition

"Let food be thy medicine and medicine be thy food" — *Hippocrates*. Proper nutrition is the foundation of a naturopathic practice, and food is used for both health promotion and disease prevention. NDs recommend diets individualized to each patient, though typically this means a balanced whole foods diet rich in fruits, vegetables, whole grains, legumes, wild-caught fish, lean animal proteins, and whole dairy products. To maximize nutritional value and minimize environmental impact, foods are considered best in their natural state, obtained locally, and eaten seasonally. NDs recognize how difficult and complex dietary changes may be, and assist patients through these changes by providing specific individualized recommendations, as well as educational materials and resources.

There is overwhelming evidence that unhealthy eating habits significantly increase the risks for morbidity and mortality. The Center for Disease Control and Prevention (CDC) determined that poor diet and physical inactivity caused 15.2% of all deaths in the United States in the year 2000, and may soon overtake tobacco as the leading cause of death.[22] It has been estimated that better nutrition could reduce the costs of heart disease, cancer, stroke, and diabetes by an estimated $71 billion each year.[23] Obesity is also at an unprecedented high in the United States. In 2009, the CDC reported that 66% of American adults, 17% of children age 12 to 19, and 19% of children age 6 to 11 years are overweight or obese.[24] The general dietary recommendations and follow-up strategies that NDs use with their patients could have a significant impact on both chronic disease and obesity. It has been well established that diets high in fruits and vegetables are associated with decreased risk for chronic disease.[25] In addition, fruits and vegetables are generally low in calories, thereby supporting healthy weight management.[26] NDs may also prescribe special diets such as the elimination diet, anti-inflammatory diet, and hypoallergenic diet. These diets have a long history of traditional use in naturopathic practice, but more research is needed in these areas to better determine clinical indications and efficacy. In one such study, the elimination diet was found to ameliorate clinical signs of inflammation in patients with rheumatoid arthritis (RA), and augment the beneficial effect of fish oil supplementation.[27]

The ultimate goal of naturopathic medicine is to optimize wellness by encouraging a healthy diet and lifestyle, but NDs may prescribe nutritional supplements if a specific deficiency is found or for certain conditions.[28] Studies have shown not only the benefits of nutritional supplementation in promoting health and preventing disease, but also the potential health care cost savings. One such study found the daily use of multivitamins containing folic acid and zinc by all women of childbearing age, and the daily use of vitamin E by those older than 50 years could save nearly $20 billion annually in hospital charges related to heart disease, birth defects, and low weight premature births.[29] There is much ongoing research in the area of nutritional supplements at both conventional and naturopathic institutions.[30]

Behavioral Change

NDs emphasize that to live healthily, one must work at it daily. Support is offered by NDs in the form of basic counseling, lifestyle modification, hypnotherapy, meditation, biofeedback, and stress management. NDs may also lead group classes in lifestyle modifications and stress management, helping foster community and connectedness for patients and physicians as they share and gain knowledge together. This holistic approach to healing acknowledges the importance of treating patients in the totality of their mind, body, and spirit. For NDs, it is essential to spend quality time listening to the patient to gain an understanding of how they live and to strengthen the physician-patient relationship. There is overwhelming evidence that effective physician-patient communication is associated with improved patient health outcomes.[31,32]

A review of mindfulness research concluded that cultivating an enhanced mindful approach to living is associated with decreases in emotional distress, increases in positive states of mind, and an improvement in quality of life. Mindfulness practice was also found to positively influence the brain, the autonomic nervous system, stress hormones, the immune system, and health behaviors, including eating, sleeping, and substance use.[33] Additional information about mindfulness research is offered in another article of this issue.

Hydrotherapy

Hydrotherapy is the external or internal use of water in any of its forms (water, ice, steam) for health promotion or treatment of disease. Hydrotherapy was used widely in ancient cultures, including Egypt, Persia, China, India, and Israel, before it was well established as the traditional European water cure.[34] Many of the treatments can be applied at home, making them cost effective and participatory for the patient.

Numerous studies have examined potential immunomodulatory effects of hydrotherapy treatments, with promising results. A study testing the immune effects of cold water therapy in cancer patients found statistically significant increases in white blood cell counts including neutrophils, lymphocytes, and monocytes, in subjects post treatment compared with pretreatment values.[35] In another study, repeated cold water stimulations in patients with chronic obstructive pulmonary disease (COPD) reduced the frequency of infections, increased lymphocyte counts, modulated interleukin expression, and improved subjective well-being.[36]

Numerous studies have also evaluated various hydrotherapy techniques for the treatment of specific conditions such as RA, osteoarthritis, wound management, hemorrhoids, varicose veins, and chronic heart failure.[37–41] Hydrotherapy was generally found to be beneficial and safe for these conditions, but broad conclusions are not warranted due to sample size limitations and inconsistent methodologies. A meta-analysis of hydrotherapy for the treatment of fibromyalgia syndrome found moderate evidence that hydrotherapy has short-term beneficial effects on pain and health-related quality of life (HRQOL).[42] A recent Cochrane review on nasal saline irrigations for chronic rhinosinusitis found evidence that nasal lavage relieves symptoms, helps as an adjunct to treatment, and is well tolerated by most patients. There were no significant side effects reported.[43] More research on hydrotherapy is indicated due to the promising preliminary findings in these areas.

Homeopathy

Homeopathy is a healing system that was created more than 200 years ago by a German physician, Samuel Hahnemann. Homeopathy is based on a central theory known as The Similia Principle. Substances made from plants, minerals, or animals, which are known to cause symptoms similar to a certain disease, are given to patients in an extremely diluted form. Homeopathic remedies are believed to stimulate autoregulatory and self-healing processes.[44] Remedies are selected by matching a patient's symptoms, based on taking a finely detailed history, with symptoms produced by the substances in healthy individuals. Homeopathy is extensively used worldwide by homeopaths, MDs, DOs, NDs, and veterinarians. Across Europe, approximately a quarter of the population uses homeopathy, and depending on the country, from 20% to 85% of all general practitioners either use homeopathy in their practices or refer their patients to homeopaths.[45]

There are more than 200 clinical trials testing the efficacy of homeopathic treatments, many of which have led to positive results. However, an inconsistency in methods, limitations in sample sizes, as well as a lack of testing for single conditions restricts pooling these results. A review evaluated the effectiveness of homeopathy in the fields of immunoallergology and common inflammatory diseases. The evidence collectively demonstrates that in some conditions homeopathy shows significant promise, for example, *Galphimia glauca* for the treatment of allergic oculorhinitis. Classic individualized homeopathy showed potential for the treatment of otitis, fibromyalgia, and possibly upper respiratory tract infections and allergic complaints. A general weakness of the evidence is scarcity of independent confirmation of reported trials and conflicting results. The investigators concluded that, considering homeopathic medicines are safe, they are a possible treatment option for upper airway infections, otitis, allergic rhinitis, and asthma.[46]

Several other clinical trials on homeopathic medicines show promise as well. One trial evaluated homeopathic medicines for minimizing the adverse effects of cancer treatments, and found preliminary data in support of the efficacy of topical calendula ointment in the prevention of radiotherapy-induced dermatitis, and Traumeel S mouthwash for chemotherapy-induced stomatitis. The medicines did not cause any serious adverse effect or interact with conventional treatment.[47] A Norwegian multicenter outcomes study found that 7 out of 10 patients visiting a homeopath reported a meaningful improvement in their main complaint 6 months after the initial consultation.[48] Given these positive findings, as well as the rich history and widespread use of homeopathy, further research in this area is indicated.

Botanical Medicine

Traditional medicine has been used in communities for thousands of years. According to the World Health Organization, herbal treatments are the most popular form of traditional medicine.[49] In developing countries, 80% of the population depends exclusively on medicinal plants for primary health care.[50] NDs use herbal preparations in the form of teas, tinctures, poultices, balms, baths, elixirs, compresses, oils, syrups, suppositories, and capsules. NDs prescribe and prepare herbal remedies based on the uniqueness of each patient and their presenting symptoms. Organic and wild harvested herbs are used if available. A growing body of research supports the efficacy and safety of various herbs for preventing and treating many health conditions.[7]

A Cochrane review of herbal medicine for low back pain found strong evidence that *Harpagophytum procumbens* (devil's claw) reduced pain better than placebo, and moderate evidence that *Salix alba* (white willow bark) and *Capsicum frutescens* (cayenne) reduced pain better than placebo in short-term trials. However, the investigators reported that the quality of reporting in these trials was generally poor, and that additional trials testing these herbal medicines against standard treatments are needed, particularly for long-term use.[51] In another Cochrane review, *Crataegus laevigata* (hawthorn leaf, flower and fruit) extract was found to provide a significant benefit in symptom control and physiologic outcomes as an adjunctive therapy for chronic heart failure. All 14 trials included in the review were double-blind, placebo-controlled randomized controlled trials (RCTs).[52] A Cochrane review of *Hypericum perforatum* (St John's wort) for the treatment of depression concluded that *Hypericum perforatum* extracts: (a) are superior to placebo in patients with major depression; (b) are similarly effective as standard antidepressants; and (c) have fewer side effects than standard antidepressants. All studies included were double-blind RCTs. However, the association of country of origin and precision with effects sizes complicated the interpretation.[53] The use of dietary supplements and primary care is explored further in another article of this issue.

Naturopathic Physical Medicine

Since the founding of naturopathy in the early twentieth century, physical medicine modalities have been an integral component of naturopathic treatments. Naturopathic physical medicine is the therapeutic use of physiotherapy, therapeutic exercise, massage, energy work, naturopathic manipulation, and hydrotherapy. This practice is distinct from that of chiropractic, physical therapy, and physical rehabilitation.[7] Although it encompasses a broad range of treatment modalities, most are used for musculoskeletal conditions, such as injury and pain.

Research on naturopathic physical modalities is limited, results have been inconsistent. A systematic review of low-intensity pulsed ultrasonography for the healing of fractures concluded that, although overall results are promising, the evidence is moderate to low in quality and provides conflicting results. The investigators recommend large, blinded trials, directly addressing patient-important outcomes, such as return to function.[54] A Cochrane review of therapeutic ultrasound for treating patellofemoral pain syndrome determined that no conclusion could be made due to poor reporting of the therapeutic application of the ultrasound and low methodological quality of the trials included.[55] A Cochrane review of transcutaneous electrical nerve stimulation (TENS) for chronic pain produced similarly questionable results. The investigators reported that published literature on the subject lacks the methodological rigor needed to make confident assessments of the role of TENS in chronic pain management, and that large multicenter RCTs of TENS are needed.[56]

NATUROPATHIC RESEARCH

Much complementary and alternative (CAM) research to date has focused on single modalities, specific supplements, and particular constituents of herbs. This type of research is taken out of context of the larger CAM medical system in which it is actually used.[57] The optimal research model used for evaluating naturopathic interventions must allow for individualized, multifaceted treatment strategies and potentially synergistic effects.[58] Whole systems research (WSR) is an emerging research paradigm that may provide a better assessment of CAM therapies than classic RCTs, which attempt to determine the single best treatment for all patients. The goal of WSR is to evaluate treatments, products, specific modalities, and techniques within the context of the unique medical system in which they are used. Fundamental to WSR is developing appropriate study designs and analysis strategies for whole systems of medicine, recognizing the individuality of treatments and the participatory role of patients, emphasizing the health care environment and physician-patient interactions, including outcome measures based on patient-held values and individualized end points, and further developing a common understanding of the CAM models being studied. WSR is nonhierarchical, cyclical, adaptive, and holds qualitative and quantitative methods in equal esteem.[57,58]

The Naturopathic Medical Research Agenda was a National Center for Complementary and Alternative Medicine (NCCAM)-funded project spanning from 2002 to 2004, which developed recommendations for the direction and emphasis of naturopathic research through 2010. Participants included more than 1200 individuals, representing a range of scientific and clinical backgrounds from leading naturopathic faculty to conventional physician scientists. Two priority populations were identified during these sessions, type 2 diabetes and elderly life stage. For both of these populations, the goal is to compare naturopathic medical care to conventional care in large controlled trials. Specific approaches to naturopathic research were also identified, which include: (1) design and implement whole-practice research protocols focusing on naturopathic medicine as a primary care practice for both prioritized populations; (2) continue to research components of naturopathic medicine to include single agents for a specified diagnosis and mechanism of action studies; and (3) perform contextual research through observational studies, and study aspects of the practice of naturopathic medicine such as the patient-practitioner interaction and its integration with the larger medical system.[59] Participating naturopathic medical schools are in the process of performing this research, and studies are at various stages of completion.[1,60,61]

There are several other current research projects, both federally and privately funded, at naturopathic medical schools in the United States and Canada. The NCCAM and The Canadian Institutes of Health Research (CIHR) are substantial funding agencies for these projects. Examples of current research include a matched controlled outcomes study comparing integrated care to conventional care for the treatment of cancer (Bastyr University and Fred Hutchinson Cancer Research Center), a pilot study evaluating the effects of magnet therapy for carpal tunnel syndrome (National College of Naturopathic Medicine), and a pragmatic randomized clinical trial of naturopathic medicine's ability to treat and prevent cardiovascular disease (Canadian College of Naturopathic Medicine).[1,60,61]

INTEGRATIVE PATIENT CARE

Goals of naturopathic medicine parallel those of family medicine in providing for and maintaining the well-being of both the patient and the health care system as a whole. Collaboration between conventional and naturopathic communities is growing as state licensing and insurance credentialing expands, and as the general public becomes more knowledgeable about CAM therapies.[62,63] Patients are increasingly seeking out NDs for many reasons, including wanting a holistic approach that addresses the root of the problem, wanting more time and attention, having not been helped by conventional care, and having had a previous positive experience with an ND.[64] Many of the conditions for which patients see licensed NDs are the same as the conditions for which they see conventional physicians.[20] For those who choose integrative medicine, comanagement of care and referral mechanisms will ensure optimally safe and effective patient care for several reasons. NDs are trained in potential drug/herb interactions and can provide educational support to patients and physicians. Naturopathic care may also reduce the need for some prescriptive drugs, and collaboration between the prescribing physician and the ND will be critical in determining medication dosing. NDs can also offer nutritional support around surgery and other procedures to reduce recovery time and potential complications. NDs are well trained in identifying potentially life-threatening situations and medical conditions that are beyond their scope of practice. Collaborative referral systems would provide continuity of care, comprehensive treatment, and optimal long-term patient management.

There are several integrative clinics nationwide that employ both NDs and MDs, and at least 20 hospitals that staff NDs. One such integrative clinic is Cedarburg Women's Health Center, located in Cedarburg, Wisconsin. The clinic was established by Janice Alexander, MD to provide primary care with prevention at the forefront. Michele

Nickels, ND joined the practice to offer patients an integrative approach to health. The collaboration has been beneficial to both the patients and physicians involved. Patients have seen that both types of medicine are needed for optimal health, and that each philosophy of medicine needs to be practiced by specialists. Dr Alexander has experienced how knowledgeable NDs are regarding primary care, and has seen substantial results from naturopathic treatments in her patients. Dr Nickels respects the expertise of Dr Alexander, and has significantly benefited from her mentorship. Discussion of patient cases has been mutually beneficial. Their patients agree that this type of medical care is at the forefront of primary care medicine.

Dr Nickels also runs a private practice, Integrative Family Wellness Center, located in Brookfield, Wisconsin. The clinic offers conventional family medicine as well as naturopathic medicine, chiropractic care, acupuncture, and manual therapy. Because of their holistic approach to health care and the additional time and attention provided to patients, the clinic has doubled in size in 1 year. Dr Nickels emphasizes that patients want this type of primary care, and envisions health care moving in this direction as people become more educated and demand having a choice of treatment options (permission from Michele Nickels, July 2009).

Another integrative clinic, located in Lokahi, Hawaii, is a partnership between Lokahi Health Center, the private practice of Michael Traub, ND, and Pacifica Integrative Skin Wellness Institute, the dermatologic private practice of Monica Scheel, MD. There is much mutual referral between the 2 businesses. Dr Traub's patients have access to the expertise of a board-certified dermatologist, and Dr Scheel's patients have access to NDs who can address concerns that go beyond their dermatologic conditions (permission from Michael Traub, July 2009).

RESOURCES

For more information, patients and physicians can go to the American Association of Naturopathic Physicians, the national association for licensed NDs, at http://www.naturopathic.org/. Additional local resources may be obtained from state naturopathic associations. The Web sites of accredited naturopathic medical schools (see **Table 2**) provide information specific to naturopathic education. There are also several texts that offer information on the practice of naturopathic medicine and its related modalities (**Box 3**). Key clinical recommendations are listed in **Table 3**.

Box 3
Suggested reading

1. *Textbook of naturopathic medicine* (2-volume set), Third Edition. Joseph E. Pizzorno Jr, ND, Michael T. Murray, ND

2. *Natural medicines comprehensive database.* Jeff M. Jellin, PharmD

3. *Woman's encyclopedia of natural medicine.* Tori Hudson, ND

4. *An Encyclopedia of natural healing for children and infants.* Mary Bove, ND

5. *Plant medicine in practice*: Using the teachings of John Bastyr. William Mitchell, ND. Elsevier Science; 2003

6. *Herbal medicine from the heart of the earth.* Sharol Tilgner, ND

7. *Feeding the whole family.* Cynthia Lair

8. *Anti-inflammation diet and recipe book.* Jessica Black, ND

Table 3
Key clinical recommendations

Recommendation	Strength of Recommendation	Reference(s)
The elimination diet improves clinical signs of inflammation in RA, and augments the beneficial effect of fish oil supplementation	B	27
Daily use of multivitamins containing folic acid and zinc by women of childbearing age, and the daily use of vitamin E by those older than 50 years reduces heart disease, birth defects, and low weight premature births.	A	29
A "mindful" approach to living is associated with decreases in emotional distress, increases in positive states of mind, and an improvement in quality of life	A	33
Cold water therapy increases white blood cell counts in cancer patients	B	35
Cold water stimulations reduce frequency of infection, increase lymphocyte counts, modulate interleukin expression, and improve subjective well-being in COPD	B	36
Hydrotherapy has short-term beneficial effects on pain and HRQOL in fibromyalgia syndrome	A	42
Nasal irrigation for chronic rhinosinusitis relieves symptoms and augments standard treatment	A	43
Classic individualized homeopathy shows potential for the treatment of otitis, fibromyalgia, and possibly upper respiratory tract infections and allergic complaints	B	46
Topical calendula ointment minimizes the adverse effects of radiotherapy-induced dermatitis, and Traumeel S mouthwash minimizes the adverse effects of chemotherapy-induced stomatitis	B	47
Harpagophytum procumbens (devil's claw), Salix alba (white willow bark), and Capsicum frutescens (cayenne) reduce low back pain better than placebo	B	51
Crataegus laevigata (hawthorn leaf, flower and fruit) extract provides benefit in symptom control and physiologic outcomes as an adjunctive treatment for chronic heart failure	A	52
Hypericum perforatum (St John's wort) extracts are superior to placebo and similar to antidepressants for major depression, with fewer side effects	A	53
Low-intensity pulsed ultrasonography may benefit the healing of fractures	B	54
Therapeutic ultrasound may benefit patellofemoral pain syndrome	C	55
TENS may aid in chronic pain management.	C	56
Collaboration between NDs and MDs has potential benefit for patients	C	62,63

Abbreviations: COPD, chronic obstructive pulmonary disease; HRQOL, health-related quality of life; RA, rheumatoid arthritis; TENS, transcutaneous electrical nerve stimulation.

ACKNOWLEDGMENTS

The work presented here was carried out while Drs Fleming and Gutknecht were Primary Care Research Fellows supported by a National Research Service Award (T32HP10010) from the Health Resources and Services Administration to the University of Wisconsin Department of Family Medicine. Michael Fleming, MD and Eric Yarnell, ND provided assistance in editing this manuscript.

REFERENCES

1. Bastyr University. Available at: http://www.bastyr.edu/education/naturopath/degree/training.asp. Accessed June 29, 2009.
2. The American Association of Naturopathic Physicians. Available at: http://www.naturopathic.org/content.asp?pl=16&contentid=16. Accessed June 30, 2009.
3. Kirchfeld F, Boyle W. Nature doctors: pioneers in naturopathic medicine. Portland, Oregon: Medicina Biologica; 1994.
4. Zeff J, Snider P, Pizzorno JE. Section I: philosophy of natural medicine. In: The textbook of natural medicine. vol. 1. 3rd edition. St Louis (MO): Churchill Livingstone Elsevier; 2006. p. 27–39.
5. Cavaliere C. World news. Naturopathic profession growing rapidly in US and Canada. HerbalGram 2007;76:22–4.
6. Poorman D, Kim L, Mittman P. Naturopathic medical education: where conventional, complementary, and alternative medicine meet. Complement Health Pract Rev 2002;7(2):99–109.
7. LaMont S, Quinn S, Donovan P, et al. Naturopathic medicine: primary care for the 21st century. Washington, DC: American Association of Naturopathic Physicians. p. 1–32.
8. Association of Accredited Naturopathic Medical Colleges. Available at: http://www.aanmc.org/. Accessed June 29, 2009.
9. Neall J, Hudson T. Naturopathic medicine residency programs. Alternative Complement Ther 2002;8(2):114–6.
10. Albert DP, Butar FB. Diffusion of naturopathic state licensing in the United States and Canada. Complement Health Pract Rev 2004;9(3):193–207.
11. North American Board of Naturopathic Examiners. Available at: http://www.nabne.org/. Accessed June 30, 2009.
12. Washington Association of Naturopathic Physicians. Available at: http://www.wanp.org/mc/page.do?sitePageId=58070&orgId=wanp. Accessed June 30, 2009.
13. Eisenberg DM, Cohen MH, Hrbek A, et al. Credentialing complementary and alternative medical providers. Ann Intern Med 2002;137(12):965–73.
14. Lafferty WE, Tyree PT, Bellas AS, et al. Insurance coverage and subsequent utilization of complementary and alternative medicine providers. Am J Manag Care 2006;12(7):397–404.
15. Barnes PM, Bloom B, Nahin RL. Complementary and alternative medicine use among adults and children: United States, 2007. U.S. Department of Health and Human Services Centers for Disease Control and Prevention 2008;12:1–24.
16. Albert DP, Martinez D. The supply of naturopathic physicians in the United States and Canada continues to increase. Complement Health Pract Rev 2006;11(2):120–2.
17. Albert DP, Butar FB. Distribution, concentration, and health care implications of naturopathic physicians in the United States. Complement Health Pract Rev 2004;9(2):103–17.

18. Weber W, Taylor JA, McCarty RL, et al. Frequency and characteristics of pediatric and adolescent visits in naturopathic medical practice. Pediatrics 2007;120(1):e142–6.

19. Boon HS, Cherkin DC, Erro J, et al. Practice patterns of naturopathic physicians: results from a random survey of licensed practitioners in two US states. BMC Complement Altern Med 2004;4:14.

20. Cherkin DC, Deyo RA, Sherman KJ, et al. Characteristics of visits to licensed acupuncturists, chiropractors, massage therapists, and naturopathic physicians. J Am Board Fam Pract 2002;15(6):463–72.

21. Weber W, Newmark S. Complementary and alternative medical therapies for attention-deficit/hyperactivity disorder and autism. Pediatr Clin North Am 2007; 54(6):983–1006, xii.

22. Mokdad AH, Marks JS, Stroup DF, et al. Actual causes of death in the United States, 2000. JAMA 2004;291(10):1238–45.

23. Frazao E. High costs of poor eating patterns in the United States. In: America's eating habits: changes and consequences, vol. 750. Washington, DC: U.S. Department of Agriculture; 1999. p. 5–32.

24. Centers for Disease Control and Prevention. Available at: http://www.cdc.gov/ nchs/fastats/overwt.htm. Accessed June 30, 2009.

25. US Department of Health and Human Services, US department of agriculture. Dietary guidelines for Americans. Washington, DC: US Government Printing Office; 2005:34. Available at: http://www.health.gov/dietaryguidelines. Accessed June 30, 2009.

26. Rolls BJ, Ello-Martin JA, Tohill BC. What can intervention studies tell us about the relationship between fruit and vegetable consumption and weight management? Nutr Rev 2004;62(1):1–17.

27. Adam O, Beringer C, Kless T, et al. Anti-inflammatory effects of a low arachidonic acid diet and fish oil in patients with rheumatoid arthritis. Rheumatol Int 2003; 23(1):27–36.

28. Lam J, Szmitko PE. Naturopathy: complementary or rudimentary medicine? Univ Toronto Med J 2002;80(1):63–5.

29. Bendich A, Mallick R, Leader S. Potential health economic benefits of vitamin supplementation. West J Med 1997;166(5):306.

30. National Center for Complementary and Alternative Medicine (NCCAM). Available at: http://nccam.nih.gov/research/extramural/awards/2008/. Accessed July 19, 2009.

31. Kaplan SH, Greenfield S, Ware JE Jr. Assessing the effects of physician-patient interactions on the outcomes of chronic disease. Med Care 1989;27(Suppl 3): S110–27.

32. Stewart MA. Effective physician-patient communication and health outcomes: a review. Can Med Assoc J 1995;152(9):1423–33.

33. Greeson JM. Mindfulness research update: 2008. Complement Health Pract Rev 2009;14(1):10.

34. Muir M. The healing power of water. Alternative Complement Ther 1998;4(6): 384–91.

35. Kuehn G. Sequential hydrotherapy improves the immune response of cancer patients. In: Mizrahi A, Fulder S, Sheinman N, editors. Potentiating health and the crisis of the immune system: integrative approaches to the prevention and treatment of modern diseases. New York: Plenum Press; 1997. p. 129–37.

36. Goedsche K, Forster M, Kroegel C, et al. Repeated cold water stimulations (hydrotherapy according to Kneipp) in patients with COPD. Forsch Komplementmed 2007;14(3):158–66.

37. Hammond A. Rehabilitation in rheumatoid arthritis: a critical review. Musculoskeletal Care 2004;2(3):135–51.
38. Silva LE, Valim V, Pessanha AP, et al. Hydrotherapy versus conventional land-based exercise for the management of patients with osteoarthritis of the knee: a randomized clinical trial. Phys Ther 2008;88(1):12–21.
39. McCulloch J. Physical modalities in wound management: ultrasound, vasopneumatic devices and hydrotherapy. Ostomy Wound Manage 1995;41(5):30–2, 34, 36-7.
40. MacKay D. Hemorrhoids and varicose veins: a review of treatment options. Altern Med Rev 2001;6(2):126–40.
41. Michalsen A, Lüdtke R, Bühring M, et al. Thermal hydrotherapy improves quality of life and hemodynamic function in patients with chronic heart failure. Am Heart J 2003;146(4):728–33.
42. Langhorst J, Musial F, Klose P, et al. Efficacy of hydrotherapy in fibromyalgia syndrome—a meta-analysis of randomized controlled clinical trials. Rheumatology (Oxford) 2009;48(9):1155–9.
43. Harvey R, Hannan SA, Badia L, et al. Nasal saline irrigations for the symptoms of chronic rhinosinusitis. Cochrane Database Syst Rev 2007;(3):CD006394.
44. Jonas WB, Kaptchuk TJ, Linde K. A critical overview of homeopathy. Ann Intern Med 2003;138(5):393–9.
45. Medhurst R. The use of homeopathy around the world. J Aust Tradit Med Soc 2004;10:153.
46. Bellavite P, Chirumbolo S, Magnani P, et al. Effectiveness of homeopathy in immunology and inflammation disorders: a literature overview of clinical studies. Homeopath Heritage 2008;33(3):35–57.
47. Kassab S, Cummings M, Berkovitz S, et al. Homeopathic medicines for adverse effects of cancer treatments. Cochrane Database Syst Rev 2009;(2): CD004845.
48. Steinsbekk A, Lüdtke R. Patients' assessments of the effectiveness of homeopathic care in Norway: a prospective observational multicentre outcome study. Homeopathy 2005;94(1):10–6.
49. WHO Traditional Medicine. Available at: http://www.who.int/mediacentre/fact sheets/fs134/en/. Accessed June 9, 2009.
50. Agra MF, Freitas PF, Barbosa-Filho JM. Synopsis of the plants known as medicinal and poisonous in northeast Brazil. Rev Bras Farmacogn 2007;17: 114–40.
51. Gagnier JJ, van Tulder MW, Berman B, et al. Herbal medicine for low back pain: a Cochrane review. Spine (Phila Pa 1976) 2007;32(1):82–92.
52. Pittler MH, Guo R, Ernst E. Hawthorn extract for treating chronic heart failure. Cochrane Database Syst Rev 2008;(1):CD005312.
53. Linde K, Berner MM, Kriston L. St John's Wort for major depression. Cochrane Database Syst Rev 2008;(4):CD000448.
54. Busse JW, Kaur J, Mollon B, et al. Low intensity pulsed ultrasonography for fractures: systematic review of randomised controlled trials. BMJ 2009;338: b351.
55. Brosseau L, Casimiro L, Robinson V, et al. Therapeutic ultrasound for treating patellofemoral pain syndrome. Cochrane Database Syst Rev 2001;(4): CD003375.
56. Nnoaham KE, Kumbang J. Transcutaneous electrical nerve stimulation (TENS) for chronic pain. Cochrane Database Syst Rev 2008;(3):CD003222.

57. Ritenbaugh C, Verhoef M, Fleishman S, et al. Whole systems research: a discipline for studying complementary and alternative medicine. Altern Ther Health Med 2003;9(4):32–6.
58. Verhoef MJ, Lewith G, Ritenbaugh C, et al. Complementary and alternative medicine whole systems research: beyond identification of inadequacies of the RCT. Complement Ther Med 2005;13(3):206–12.
59. Standish LJ, Calabrese C, Snider P. The naturopathic medical research agenda: the future and foundation of naturopathic medical science. J Altern Complement Med 2006;12(3):341–5.
60. National College of Naturopathic Medicine: Helfgott Research Institute. Available at: http://helfgott.org/projects.php. Accessed July 6, 2009.
61. Canadian College of Naturopathic Medicine. Available at: http://www.ccnm.edu/?q=current_research. Accessed July 6, 2009.
62. Dunne N, Benda W, Kim L, et al. Naturopathic medicine: what can patients expect? J Fam Pract 2005;54(12):1067–72.
63. Smith MJ, Logan AC. Naturopathy. Med Clin North Am 2002;86(1):173–84.
64. Leung B, Verhoef M. Survey of parents on the use of naturopathic medicine in children—characteristics and reasons. Complement Ther Clin Pract 2008;14(2):98–104.

Integrating Sustainability and Health Care

Rian J. Podein, MD[a],*, Michael T. Hernke, PhD[b]

KEYWORDS

• Sustainability • Health care • The Natural Step

Concerns regarding sustainability are at the forefront of societal awareness. Globally, unsustainable development has contributed to ecological degradation and human suffering while compromising the ability of ecosystems and social institutions to support human life. The United States health care system and its institutions are significant contributors to unsustainable development, but leaders of change are emerging from the health care arena. Health professionals, including primary care providers, are poised to serve as models for sustainability and to facilitate necessary transformation toward more sustainable practices. Embracing an objective definition of sustainability within a practical framework and then acting toward the goal of sustainability are crucial components for success.

DEFINING SUSTAINABILITY

In 1987, the United Nations (UN) published a report that provided guiding principles for sustainable development as it is generally understood today. That is: "Sustainable development is development that meets the needs of the present without compromising the ability of future generations to meet their own needs."[1] The Natural Step (TNS), a nonprofit organization, puts this philosophic definition into practice in its first-order principles for guiding society. These include four principles known as "system conditions," which have been reviewed elsewhere and are described as follows[2]:

In a sustainable society, nature is not subject to systematically increasing

1. concentrations of substances extracted from the Earth's crust,
2. concentrations of substances produced by society,

---

[a] Department of Family Medicine, University of Wisconsin School of Medicine and Public Health, 1100 Delaplaine Court, Madison, WI 53715, USA
[b] Department of Operations & Information Management, School of Business, University of Wisconsin-Madison, 975 University Avenue, Madison, WI 53706, USA
* Corresponding author.
E-mail address: Rian.Podein@fammed.wisc.edu (R.J. Podein).

Prim Care Clin Office Pract 37 (2010) 137–147
doi:10.1016/j.pop.2009.09.011
0095-4543/10/$ – see front matter © 2010 Elsevier Inc. All rights reserved.

3. degradation by physical means; and
4. In that society, people are not subject to conditions that systematically undermine their capacity to meet their needs.

The TNS principles for a sustainable society make it possible to objectively diagnose the causes of unsustainable development, including those related to health care.

The Natural Step System Condition One: In a Sustainable Society, Nature is Not Subject to Systematically Increasing Concentrations of Substances Extracted from the Earth's Crust

Society mines and disperses materials at a faster rate than they are redeposited back into the Earth's crust. Globally, fossil fuels are extracted and burned in enormous quantities every year: more than 1.2 cubic miles of oil, 3.5 billion metric tons of coal, and 100 trillion cubic feet of natural gas.[3] The United States health care sector spends over $5 billion dollars annually for energy, and ranks second only to the food service industry for energy consumption.[4] United States hospitals use twice the energy of other buildings and of comparable European hospitals.[5] The use of fossil fuels is directly responsible for the potentially catastrophic accumulation of greenhouse gases and global climate change.[6] Climate change is known to affect human health via a multitude of pathways, including temperature-related illnesses and deaths, extreme weather, air pollution, allergic diseases, infectious diseases, malnutrition, and displaced populations.[7,8] Global climate change has been conservatively estimated to be responsible for 150,000 deaths annually.[9] On top of this problem, violation of the first principle leads to systematically increasing concentrations of metals and mineral residues in natural systems, such as arsenic in drinking water; cadmium in kidneys; lead in children; mercury in fish, pregnant women, and human nervous tissue; and phosphates in lakes. Meanwhile concern is growing about potential, but so far unknown, effects from increasing concentrations of such metals as zinc and silver.

Practice pearl #1
Consider completing the attached energy conservation checklist from the Teleosis Institute, a program of Practice Greenhealth (**Fig. 1**). With improvement and refinement of your practices, your checklist score will increase and your contribution to unsustainable energy consumption, global climate change, and other harmful effects will decrease.

The Natural Step System Condition Two: In a Sustainable Society, Nature is Not Subject to Systematically Increasing Concentrations of Substances Produced by Society

Substances that society produces leak into natural systems faster than natural processes can break them down. The United States alone has developed, distributed, and discarded more than 80,000 chemicals into the environment over the past 50 years with the majority not tested for potential toxicities.[10] Two notable examples within health care are (1) dioxins that have been discharged over long periods via medical waste incineration and (2) increasing concentrations of pharmaceuticals within United States streams and supplies of drinking water, a more recent concern.[11,12] Dioxin is a known human carcinogen that persists in the environment for decades. Pharmaceuticals, on the other hand, are being prescribed in increasing quantities and are either excreted or discarded to such an extent that they are accumulating faster than they degrade. Unlike the chemically persistent organic products like dioxin, pharmaceuticals are considered "pseudopersistent" because of their continuous presence in the environment and have been named by the Environmental

ENERGY CONSERVATION

ENERGY ASSESSMENT AND HVAC MAINTENANCE	Possible Points	A) Does it apply to you?	B) Your Possible Points	C) Did you do it?	D) Your Score
Have your energy provider conduct a free audit of your facility's energy use to provide you with specific suggestions to conserve energy.	2				
Review the assessment and this checklist annually to identify additional opportunities to improve energy savings.	2				
Conduct monthly energy inspections and offer incentives to employees in return for energy saving practices.	2				
EQUIPMENT	Possible Points	A) Does it apply to you?	B) Your Possible Points	C) Did you do it?	D) Your Score
Use office equipment with energy saving features. When making new purchases, look for computers, copiers, printers, with better Energy Efficient Ratings.	2				
Set computer defaults to automatically turn off idle monitors and printers.	1				
Plug office equipment into a time switch to turn off after working hours.	1				
Replace inefficient refrigerators (usually older than ten years) with newer models that have a better Energy Efficient Rating.	4				
Convert electric hot water heaters to natural gas.	4				
Insulate pipes and hot water heaters.	3				

Fig. 1. Energy conservation checklist. (*Courtesy of* Teleosis Institute [a program of Practice Greenhealth]; Berkeley, CA; with permission.)

	Possible Points	A) Does it apply to you?	B) Your Possible Points	C) Did you do it?	D) Your Score
Use a solar water heater or preheater.	4				
Assess recycling options for end of life electronics to ensure they are disposed of safely.	3				
LIGHTING					
Replace incandescent bulbs with one of the following:					
Halogen PAR lamps	1				
Compact fluorescent bulbs	1				
Low voltage track lighting	1				
Increase efficiency of fluorescent fixture in one of the following ways:					
Put in higher efficiency lighting, such as high-pressure sodium or metal halides	2				
Replace magnetic ballasts with electronic ballasts	3				
Install T-8 or T-5 lamps	3				
Reduce the number of lamps and increase lighting efficiency by installing optical reflectors or diffusers	3				
Improve exit sign efficiency by using one of the following:					
LED exit signs	1				
Compact fluorescent bulbs in exit signs	1				
Electroluminescent exit signs	1				
Install lighting controls with one of the following:					
Movement sensors	2				
Bypass or delay timers	1				
Photocells	1				
Time clocks	1				

Fig. 1 (continued)

HEATING/ COOLING UNITS	Possible Points	A) Does it apply to you?	B) Your Possible Points	C) Did you do it?	D) Your Score
Perform regular maintenance on your HVAC (heating, ventilation and air conditioning) system. The HVAC should be regularly cleaned, replacing dirty air filters, and checked for leaks, proper pilot lighting and other problems. If leasing your facility, ask the building owner or manger to do this.	3				
Install ceiling fans.	2				
Apply window film to reduce solar heat gain.	2				
Shade sun-exposed windows and walls during the cooling season. Use awnings, sunscreens, shade trees or shrubbery.	3				
Replace or supplement an A/C system with an evaporative cooler.	2				
Install economizers on A/C to increase air circulation.	2				
Replace old A/C units with newer models that have a better Energy Efficient Rating.	4				
Convert electric heating system to a natural gas system.	4				
Install bypass timers or time clocks for the HVAC system.	1				
Replace inefficient or broken windows with double-pane, energy efficient windows.	3				
Use weatherizing and caulking to seal windows and doors.	2				
Provide shading for HVAC condenser.	1				

ENERGY SAVING PRACTICES	Possible Points	A) Does it apply to you?	B) Your Possible Points	C) Did you do it?	D) Your Score
Use task lighting where extra light is needed, rather than lighting an entire area.	1				
Rearrange workspaces to take advantage of areas with natural sunlight, and design for increased natural lighting when remodeling.	2				
Always turn off lights when leaving and post reminders.	1				

Fig. 1 (*continued*)

	Possible Points	A) Does it apply to you?	B) Your Possible Points	C) Did you do it?	D) Your Score
Dust diffusers annually for optimum light output.	1				
Set thermostat at 68° for heating and 78° for cooling. Use timing devices to turn system down after hours.	1				
Set refrigerator temperature between 38° and 42° and freezer between 0° and 5°.	1				
Use small fans and space heaters during off hours instead of heating the entire office.	1				
Close blinds and curtains (to reflect sunlight) or use ceiling fans to reduce A/C load.	1				
Seal off unused areas of the building. Block and insulate unneeded windows and other openings.	2				
When repainting building exterior and roofs, choose light colors to reflect more sunlight.	1				
Institute a formal policy to turn off equipment and lights when not in use.	1				
Maintain equipment optimum efficiency.	1				
Use the standby mode on equipment (e.g. energy saver buttons on copiers).	1				
OTHER ACTIVITIES *Please describe additional activities and assign points. This will be reviewed by GHC Team.*	Possible Points	A) Does it apply to you?	B) Your Possible Points	C) Did you do it?	D) Your Score
TOTAL					

	TOTAL of Your Possible Points	TOTAL of Your Score	SECTION SCORE
ENERGY CONSERVATION			

Fig. 1 (continued)

Protection Agency as one of the top "emerging" contaminants affecting human and ecological health.[13,14]

Contamination by synthetic chemicals has been observed in humans as early as birth with an average of 200 industrial chemicals, pesticides, and other pollutants (including dioxin) identified in the umbilical cord blood of babies born in the United States. Many of these pollutants are known to cause cancer, be toxic to the brain and nervous system, and cause birth defects or abnormal development.[15] More extensive and ongoing biomonitoring studies of the general population by the Centers for Disease Control and Prevention have made it clear that all American children and adults have ingested, inhaled, or absorbed a variety of synthetic chemicals to such a degree that detectable levels of such chemicals can be found in their blood and urine.[16]

Practice pearl #2

To learn more about dioxins and dioxin-free alternatives available in the health care setting, visit www.noharm.org.

To reduce pharmaceutical pollution, clinicians can avoid prescribing more medications than can be used, prescribe starter packs and refill packs, review and regularly reassess the patient's total consumption of medication, consider environmental impact when prescribing medications, learn more about which drugs have large environmental impacts, educate consumers about the importance of proper disposal of pharmaceutical waste, and start a medication take-back program. For more information, go to www.teleosis.org and click on "Green Pharmacy."

The Natural Step System Condition Three: In a Sustainable Society, Nature is Not Subject to Systematically Increasing Degradation by Physical Means

Society is destroying the natural environment by such activities as clear-cutting, over-harvesting, paving, irrigation, among other activities, at a rate faster then can be regenerated. Specific attention can be focused on the effects of health care on forest and freshwater ecosystem degradation. American hospitals generate 4 billion lb of waste each year, more than half of which comprises such forest products as paper and cardboard.[17] In addition, up to hundreds of thousands of gallons of water are used per year per hospital bed.[18]

Violating System Conditions 1, 2, & 3

Through violations of the first three principles, society is now depleting the Earth's natural capital and the benefits nature provides, such as clean water, food, forest products, flood control, and natural resources. According to the UN, "Human activities are putting such strain on the environment that the ability of the planet's ecosystems to sustain future generations can no longer be taken for granted."[19] The Ecological Footprint provides a measure of how much land and water area a human population requires to produce the resources it consumes and to absorb its wastes under prevailing technology.[20] The ecological footprint shows that humanity increasingly consumes more resources than the planet can regenerate. Recent calculations measure our global demand at 30% greater than supply (**Fig. 2**).[21] In other words, it now takes more than 1 year and 4 months for the Earth to regenerate what humanity uses in a single year. The United States contributes disproportionately to this global "overshoot." We would need 4.5 Earths if the global population had the average United States footprint per capita. Extrapolation from economic data suggests that the United States health care system, which comprises over 16% of United States economic activity, contributes significantly to our disproportionate ecological footprint.[22]

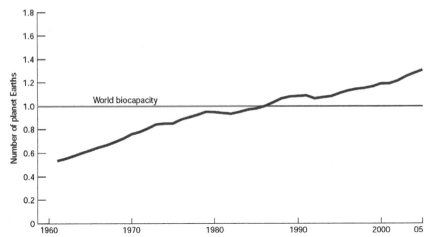

Fig. 2. Human ecological footprint (*red line*), 1961—2005. (Source: Living Planet Report 2008 — Published in October 2008 by WWF. Text and graphics copyright © 2008 WWF. All rights reserved; used with permission.)

Practice pearl #3

Go to www.footprintnetwork.org/en/index.php/GFN/page/calculators to calculate your personal ecological footprint, discover your biggest areas of resource consumption, and learn what you can do to tread more lightly on the earth.

The Natural Step System Condition Four: In That Society, People are Not Subject to Conditions That Systematically Undermine Their Capacity to Meet Their Needs

This system condition draws attention to the way in which people are using and sharing the Earth's limited resources and makes the point that sustainable development is also about the relationships within human society as they affect the health of our planet. Globally, the gap between the world's rich and poor is widening and the needs of many are being ignored. Specifically, access to health care is considered by many to be a human right and has been ratified as such within the UN Declaration of Human Rights.[23] In the United States, failure to provide guaranteed access to affordable health care has resulted in tens of millions of citizens without health insurance.[24] The lack of health insurance is a factor in making Americans less healthy and in forcing many bankruptcies, over half of which are due to illness or medical bills.[25] Furthermore, the lack of health insurance has been estimated by the Institute of Medicine to be responsible for over 18,000 adult deaths annually.[26]

Practice pearl #4

Health professionals are essential advocates in the struggle for a universal right to affordable health care. Among the multiple approaches to achieving this goal is the model based on single-payer national health insurance. To learn more about single-payer national health insurance, visit Physician's for a National Health Program at www.pnhp.org. Whatever your conclusions on single payer options, get involved and consider advocating for legislation that can increase access to affordable health care.

STEPPING TOWARD SUSTAINABILITY

Because good health is an important overarching goal for society and argued by some to be the ultimate reason for seeking sustainability, health professionals are poised to model sustainability and lead others toward more healthy outcomes.[27] In such activities as promoting peace and advocating nuclear disarmament, health professionals have had prior success using their skills to evaluate trends in global health interdependence to address problems of the twenty-first century. The new global crisis of unsustainable development necessitates similar urgent attention.

Leaders within organized medicine have responded in part by raising awareness and calling for action. Such a call for action was expressed in an editorial from the president of the American Medical Association:

> As physicians, we pledge to 'do no harm.' With that in mind, I urge you to make your practice greener in ways that are ecologically sustainable, are safe for public health and the environment, and promote good patient care.[28]

Opportunities for professional development within sustainability education and for leadership training in "sustainable medicine" have emerged. Sustainability: Step by Natural Step is an innovative on-line course developed by TNS to provide practical sustainability education and guide learners through a process of clarifying strategic approaches to real-world sustainability issues.[29] Specific to medicine and health care is the Practice Greenhealth's Teleosis Institute Leadership in Green Health Care program 8-week correspondence course, which reviews the most up-to-date theory and research behind sustainable medicine and introduces participants to the best practices for initiating green health care.[30]

Other health care industry efforts have been manifested in the emergence of such membership organizations as Practice Greenhealth, which includes hospitals, health care systems, businesses, and other stakeholders committed to applying sustainable practices in medicine; in the development of CleanMed, an annual conference for leaders in health care to accelerate the development, use, and diffusion of environmentally preferable products and practices in health care; and in the creation of the *Green Guide for Health Care*, which provides a best practices guide for sustainable building design, construction, and operations in the health care industry.

SUMMARY

Efforts within medicine and health care to mitigate violations of sustainability are commendable but only a beginning. For modern medicine, health care, and related institutions to help society advance toward a sustainable future, a clear vision and practical plan to guide such a massive transformation is desperately needed. Rather than address the many environmental and societal problems one at a time, we need to understand and approach them at the systemic level. According to Doctor Karl-Henrik Robèrt, founder of the TNS organization, three questions must be addressed to make advancements and ensure sustainability within an organization and society. Those questions are:

1. Does your organization have a definition of sustainability?
2. What is, with reference to this definition, your gap to sustainability?
3. What are you doing, at the strategic level of the organization, to bridge that gap?

Decisions should not be made until those three questions have been satisfactorily answered. Since all three questions point toward sustainability, promising solutions will emerge from decisions based on those answers, says Robèrt. Although sustainability is a global concept, a single person, organization, or industry, such as health care, can at least reduce and ultimately eliminate its contribution to the mechanisms causing harm.

ACKNOWLEDGMENTS

We are grateful for the inspiration and guidance of Dr Karl-Henrik Robèrt, The Natural Step organization, and all those leading society toward sustainability.

REFERENCES

1. World Commission on Environment and Development. Our common future. Oxford; New York: Oxford University Press; 1987.
2. Robèrt K-H, Schmidt-Bleek B, Aloisi de Larderel J, et al. Strategic sustainable development—selection, design and synergies of applied tools. J Cleaner Prod 2002;10:197–214.
3. Auerbach PS. Physicians and the environment. JAMA 2008;299(8):956–8.
4. United States Department of Energy. 2003 commercial building energy consumption survey. Available at: http://www.eia.doe.gov/emeu/recs/contents.html. Accessed January 1, 2009.
5. United States Department of Energy. Energy efficiency and renewable energy, building technologies program—commercial buildings. Available at: http://www1. eere.energy.gov/buildings/commercial/health_care.html. Accessed January 1, 2009.
6. Intergovernmental Panel on Climate Change. Working Group I. In: Climate change 2007: the physical science basis: contribution of Working Group I to the Fourth Assessment Report of the Intergovernmental Panel on Climate Change. Cambridge: Cambridge University Press; 2007. p. 135.
7. Haines A, Patz JA. Health effects of climate change. JAMA 2004;291(1):99–103.
8. Epstein PR. Climate change and human health. N Engl J Med 2005;353(14): 1433–6.
9. Anthony J, McMichael A, Campbell-Lendrum D, et al. Global climate change. In: Ezzati M, Lopez A, Roders A, editors. Comparative quantification of health risks, global and regional burden of disease attributable to selected major risk factors. Geneva (Switzerland): World Health Organization; 2004. p. 1543–650.
10. United States Government Accountability Office. Chemical regulation: options exist to improve EPA's ability to assess health risks and manage its chemical review program: Report to Congressional Requesters. GAO-05–458; 2005.
11. Kolpin DW, Furlong ET, Meyer MT, et al. Pharmaceuticals, hormones and other organic wastewater contaminants in US streams, 1999–2000: a national reconnaissance. Environ Sci Technol 2002;36(6):1202–11.
12. Donn J, Mendoza M, Pritchard J. Probe finds drugs in drinking water. Associated Press; March 9, 2008. Available at: http://www.usatoday.com/news/nation/2008-03-10-drugs-tap-water_N.htm. Accessed January 1, 2009.
13. Boehringer SK. What's the best way to dispose of medications? Pharmacist's Letter/Prescriber's Letter 2004;20(4):1–5.
14. Daughton C, Ternes T. Pharmaceuticals and personal care products in the environment: agents of subtle change? Environ Health Perspect 1999;107(Suppl 6): 907–43.
15. The pollution in newborns. Environmental working group, July 2005. Available at: http://archive.ewg.org/reports/bodyburden2/execsumm.php. Accessed January 1, 2009.

16. Centers for Disease Control and Prevention. Third national report on human exposure to environmental chemicals. Atlanta (GA): CDC; 2005. p. 1–467.
17. Gerwig K. Waste management & healthcare. In: Proceedings from the setting healthcare's environmental agenda conference. San Francisco (CA): October 16, 2000, p. 1–5. Available at: http://www.noharm.org/library/docs/SHEA_Proceedings_Waste_Management_White_Paper.pdf. Accessed January 1, 2009.
18. Practice greenhealth. Green guide for health care series, water conservation strategies. Available at: http://cms.h2e-online.org/ee/facilities/waterconserve/#HealthCareFacilityWaterUse. Accessed January 1, 2009.
19. Millennium Ecosystem Assessment. Ecosystems and human well-being: synthesis. Washington DC: Island Press; 2005. 1–137.
20. Holmberg J, Lundqvist U, Robert K-H, et al. The ecological footprint from a systems perspective of sustainability. Int J Sustain Dev World Ecol 1999;6: 17–33.
21. World wildlife fund for nature. Living planet report 2008. Hails C, Humphrey S, Loh J, et al, editors. Gland, Switzerland 2008: 1–45. Available at:http://assets.panda.org/downloads/living_planet_report_2008.pdf. Accessed January 1, 2009.
22. Organization for Economic Co-operation and Development. OECD health data 2009 - frequently requested data. Available at: http://www.oecd.org/document/16/0,3343,en_2649_34631_2085200_1_1_1_1,00.html. Accessed January 1, 2010.
23. Universal Declaration of Human Rights, G.A. res. 217A (III), U.N. Doc A/810 at 71. New York: United Nations, 1948.
24. DeNavas-Walt C, Proctor BD, Lee CH. U.S. Census Bureau, current population reports, P60-231, income, poverty, and health insurance coverage in the United States: 2005. Washington, DC: U.S. Government Printing Office; 2006.
25. Himmelstein DU, Warren E, Thorne D, et al. Illness and injury as contributors to bankruptcy. Health Aff Web Exclusive. February 2, 2005: W5-63-W5-73. DOI: 10.1377/hlthaff.W5.63.
26. Committee on the Consequences of Uninsurance. Care without coverage: too little, too late. Washington, DC: National Academies Press; 2002.
27. McMichael AJ. Population health as a primary criterion of sustainability. EcoHealth 2006;3:182–6.
28. Davis RM. Making health care greener. AMA eVoice April 24, 2008. Available at: http://www.ama-assn.org/ama/pub/category/18519.html. Accessed January 1, 2009.
29. Available at The Natural Step web site: www.naturalstep.org. Accessed September 30, 2008.
30. Available at Teleosis Institute web site: www.teleosis.org. Accessed June 13, 2009.

Integrative Care of the Mother-Infant Dyad

Jill Mallory, MD

KEYWORDS

• Integrative • Pregnancy • Nutrition • Labor • Herbs

In obstetric training, the outcome often sought is simply "healthy mother and baby," but how one gets from the moment of conception to "healthy mother and baby" is a journey that can affect the physical and mental health of a woman and her child for a lifetime. Certainly, in the western medical model, there are many pharmaceuticals and invasive procedures that can provide lifesaving shortcuts to the desired outcome, but do these high-tech interventions empower patients? Tsui and colleagues[1] found that 13% of pregnant women surveyed in an academic medical center used dietary supplements during pregnancy. Hollyer and coworkers[2] reported that 62% of pregnant women with nausea and vomiting of pregnancy used some form of integrative medicine to treat their symptoms. With the rise in popularity of integrative medicine, more and more patients are seeking more natural and interactive approaches to prenatal care and childbirth. It is essential that the physician be familiar with the safety and efficacy of these approaches.

In this article, dietary guidelines and supplementation of the pregnant patient are discussed first, because nutrition is the cornerstone of prevention and optimal outcomes. The use of alternative therapies for common complaints in pregnancy and in labor preparation is also reviewed. Lastly, the importance of continuous support during labor, and selected natural pain relief options, is discussed.

NUTRITION AND SUPPLEMENTS IN PREGNANCY
General Nutrition Needs

Nutritional counseling and knowledge in the use of dietary supplements are important aspects of prenatal care. In 2003, Glover and coworkers[3] published a study of 578 pregnant women in the eastern United States that found that 45% used herbal medicines and 20% were not even taking a prenatal vitamin. General daily nutritional needs for pregnant women are 300 additional calories, 80 g of protein, 1200 mg calcium, 30 mg of iron, 800 μg of folic acid, at least 5000 IU of vitamin D_3, and 1000 mg docosahexaenoic acid and eicosapentaenoic acid. Low-income women are especially at risk for dietary deficiencies in calcium, magnesium, and iron. It is important to not only review

---

Department of Family Medicine, School of Medicine and Public Health, University of Wisconsin, 1100 Delaplaine Court, Madison, WI 53715-1896, USA
E-mail address: jill.mallory@fammed.wisc.edu

Prim Care Clin Office Pract 37 (2010) 149–163
doi:10.1016/j.pop.2009.09.008
0095-4543/10/$ – see front matter © 2010 Elsevier Inc. All rights reserved.

a dietary history for patients to look for these components and educate them on where their diet may be lacking, but the physician should also be prepared to discuss food sources of each nutrient. It may be helpful to keep handouts in the office that list healthy food sources for each nutrient (**Box 1**).

A few other guidelines useful for pregnant women include recommendations to avoid Trans fats, simple carbohydrates, processed foods, and fish with high mercury levels. All pregnant women should be given information regarding which fish have lowest mercury levels so that they can choose wisely. The Environmental Protection Agency has a Web site with good information on fish and mercury levels (http://www.epa.gov/waterscience/fish/). Women should be encouraged to include as many fruits, vegetables, and whole grains as possible in their diets.

Iron

Anemia is a common finding on routine screening laboratories in pregnancy. Often, women require iron supplementation, because of dietary deficiency. Conventional iron supplements, such as ferrous sulfate, can cause gastrointestinal upset and frequently lead to constipation, causing many women to be noncompliant with taking them. There are some better tolerated alternatives available, although little research exists to document their efficacy.

Gentle Iron by Solgar is iron bisglycinate, which is widely available and has less gastrointestinal side effects. A few other products one may find in a health food store include Floradix liquid, an herbal preparation combined with ferrous gluconate, 10 mg/mL, dosed at 10 mL, taken three to four times daily before meals. Yellow dock tincture is an herbal preparation high in iron that is also safe in pregnancy. It is dosed at 3 droppers full three times daily. One ounce of fresh wheatgrass juice daily also safely boosts iron stores. Some patients have also used homeopathic ferrous phosphate at a dose of 30 c three times a day. Other herbs high in iron and safe to take in pregnancy include alfalfa, nettle, dandelion, and shephard's purse. Physicians should check with a trained herbalist before using other herbal forms of iron replacement (**Box 2**). Because there has been little to no research on using alternative forms of iron supplementation, the physician is advised to recheck hemoglobin levels in patients to ensure efficacy.

Box 1
Ten nutrition handouts to keep in the office

1. General nutrition guidelines in pregnancy
2. Food sources of iron
3. Food sources of magnesium
4. Food sources of calcium
5. Food sources of folic acid
6. Food sources of protein
7. Vitamin D sources and supplementation
8. Omega-3 fatty acid sources and supplementation
9. Which fish are safe in pregnancy
10. Glycemic index/glycemic load

Box 2
Herbs to avoid in pregnancy

- Agave plant (*Agave americana*)
- Aloe (dried juice) (*Aloe* spp)
- American pennyroyal herb (*Hedeoma pulegioides*)
- Andrographis herb (*Andrographis paniculata*)
- Angelica root (*Angelica archangelica, A atropurpurea, A sinensis*)
- Anise fruit (seed) (*Pimpinella anisum*)
- Arnica herb (*Arnica* spp)
- Ashwaganda root (*Withania somnifera*)
- Barberry root bark (*Berberis vulgaris*)
- Barley sprouted seed (*Hordeum vulgare*)
- Basil leaf (*Ocimum basilicum*)
- Black cohosh root (*Actaea racemosa*)
- Blessed thistle herb (*Cnicus benedictus*)
- Bloodroot (*Sanguinaria canadensis*)
- Blue cohosh root (*Caulophyllum thalictroides*)
- Borage herb (*Borago officinalis*)
- Butterbur rhizome (*Petasites hybridus*)
- Camphor distillate (*Cinnamomum camphora*)
- Canada snakeroot (*Asarum canadense*)
- Cascara sagrada bark (*Cascara sagrada*)
- Cassia bark (*Cinnamomum cassia*)
- Castor seed oil (*Ricinus communis*)
- Catnip herb (*Nepeta cataria*)
- Celery seed (*Apium graveolens*)
- Chastetree fruit (berry) (*Vitex agnus-castus*)
- Coltsfoot flower (*Tussilago farfara*)
- Comfrey leaf and root (*Symphytum officinale*)
- Dong quai root (*Angelica sinensis*)
- Ephedra herb (*Ephedra* spp)
- European pennyroyal (*Mentha pulegium*)
- False unicorn rhizome (*Chamaelirium luteum*)
- Fenugreek seed (*Trigonella foenum-graecum*)
- Feverfew herb (*Tanacetum parthenium*)
- Garlic bulb (*Allium sativum*)
- Ginger root (*Zingiber officinale*)
- Goldenseal root (*Hydrastis canadensis*)
- Guggul gum resin (*Commiphora mukul*)
- Ipecac rhizome (*Cephaelis ipecacuanha*)

- Kava root (*Piper methysticum*)
- Lemongrass herb (*Cymbopogon citrates*)
- Licorice root (*Glycyrrhiza* spp)
- Lobelia herb (*Lobelia inflata*)
- Ma huang (*Ephedra* spp)
- Mace seed (*Myristica fragrans*)
- Mandrake root (*Podophyllum peltatum*)
- Motherwort herb (*Leonurus cardiaca*)
- Mugwort herb (*Artemesia vulgaris, A lactiflora*)
- Myrrh gum resin (*Commiphora molmol, C myrrha*)
- Nutmeg seed (*Myristica fragrans*)
- Parsley leaf and root (*Petroselinum crispum*)
- Purslane herb (*Portulaca oleracea*)
- Quinine bark (*Cinchona* spp)
- Red clover flowers (*Trifolium pratense*)
- Red cedar leaf and berry (*Juniperus virginiana*)
- Rhubarb rhizome/root (*Rheum palmatum, R officinale*)
- Rosemary leaf (*Rosmarinus officinalis*)
- Saffron stigma (*Crocus sativus*)
- Sage leaf (*Salvia officinalis*)
- Senna leaf (*Senna* spp)
- Shepard's purse herb (*Capsella bursa-pastoris*)
- Tansy herb (*Tanacetum vulgare*)
- Turmeric rhizome (*Curcuma longa*)
- Uva ursi leaf (*Arctostaphylos uva-ursi*)
- Wormwood herb (*Artemisia absinthium*)
- Yarrow flowers (*Achillea millefolium*)
- Yellow jasmine herb (*Gelsemium sempervirens*)

This list gives only some common herbs and is not complete. *Data from* Low Dog T, Micozzi M. Women's health in complementary and alternative medicine: a clinical guide. 1st edition. St Louis: Elsevier; 2005.

Omega-3 fatty acids

Omega-3 fatty acid supplementation during pregnancy is necessary for almost all women in the United States, because of low dietary intake.[4] A depletion of omega-3 fats, notably docosahexaenoic acid and eicosapentaenoic acid, occurs during pregnancy because of the high demands of fetal central nervous system development.[5–7] Prenatal omega-3 fatty acid intake provides a protective effect on pregnancy outcomes. These include increasing length of gestation, and reduction in preeclampsia and cerebral palsy.[8] Data also support neurodevelopmental advantages for fetuses with increased exposure to omega-3 fats.[9,10] Fortunately, studies looking at the safety of over-the-counter fish oil capsules have found them to be virtually mercury free.[11] It is recommended that pregnant and lactating women take at least 1000 mg of docosahexaenoic acid and eicosapentaenoic acid in the form of fish oil capsules nightly, unless they are eating a fatty fish meal two to three times per week. Capsules can be kept in the refrigerator or freezer to reduce gastrointestinal side effects.

Vegetarian or vegan women can use flaxseed oil in capsules, usually two capsules daily, or freshly ground whole flaxseeds, usually 1 to 2 tablespoons daily, as a source of omega-3 fats. It should be noted that there is some evidence that flaxseed oil might decrease platelet aggregation. Whether or not this is clinically significant is unclear. There has been no association between the consumption of flax during pregnancy and increased risk of bleeding after delivery.

Vitamin D

Evidence on the importance of vitamin D in pregnant and lactating women is mounting. The old recommendations that mothers get 400 IU per day of vitamin D are no longer valid according to new data.[12–14] A recent review on vitamin D in pregnancy and lactation published in the peer reviewed journal *Breastfeeding Medicine* suggests optimal vitamin D_3 intake to be between 4000 and 6400 IU daily.[15] According to these reviewers, such supplementation provides some protection to both mother and child against a whole host of diseases, including diabetes, cardiovascular disease, rickets, and multiple cancers. There is no evidence of toxicity at these doses. There is even one recent retrospective observational analysis showing low maternal vitamin D levels to be associated with an increased rate of caesarean section.[16]

While awaiting more definitive data, it is suggested that pregnant and lactating patients take 5000 IU of vitamin D_3. This dose is cheap and widely available. There are capsule and liquid D_3 supplements on the market that contain 5000 IU in one capsule or drop.

Probiotics

One final nutritional supplement to consider during the prenatal period is probiotic supplementation. The use of live microorganisms, called probiotics, to benefit health has a long tradition of safety. Studies looking at the effects on pregnancy and children have been increasing in number over the past 10 years. In one meta-analysis, prenatal probiotic intake by mothers was associated with a decreased rate of atopic dermatitis in their children (number needed to treat equaled 12).[17] There is also some evidence to suggest that probiotic supplementation may reduce the risk of allergies in children delivered by cesarean section.[18] Because probiotics are relatively cheap and safe, it is reasonable to recommend pregnant women with a family history that puts them at high risk of having an atopic child take probiotics daily during pregnancy.

COMMON COMPLAINTS IN PREGNANCY
Round Ligament and Low Back Pain

Round ligament pain and low back pain are just two of many musculoskeletal complaints with which pregnant women present. There are many nonpharmacologic approaches. Prenatal yoga can be very soothing to the pregnant body, and poses can often be tailored to specific complaints. For example, having women tilt the pelvis forward and backward while standing can relieve round ligament discomfort. Women can also get on all fours on the floor, then arch, then relax the back rhythmically to relieve low back pain. For a complete reference on exercises in pregnancy, read *Essential Exercises for the Childbearing Year* by Elizabeth Noble.[19]

Prenatal massage is relaxing and can relieve muscular tension and spasm. One should guide patients to massage therapists specifically trained to work with pregnant women, because certain massage points may stimulate uterine contractions. Topical herbs that are safe for use during massage include camphor, cajeput oil, wintergreen oil, and eucalyptol. Women can purchase these for their own use at home or have a therapist incorporate them into the massage of painful areas. There are some essential oils that should not be used in pregnancy. Women should consult an experienced practitioner before using other essential oils.

Nausea and Vomiting of Pregnancy

Nausea and vomiting in early pregnancy, commonly called "morning sickness," is often one of the first complaints with which prenatal patients present. There are many options in treating the patient with morning sickness.[20] First-line therapy should be good hydration and the consumption of small frequent meals. Crackers or bread at the bedside for eating before rising may be helpful to some women. Peppermint tea can be added to the diet for nausea, but may exacerbate constipation. In addition to nutrition, acupuncture and acupressure are safe and effective options.[21] Ginger, vitamin B_6, and doxylamine may also be helpful.

Ginger has been studied and shown effective for morning sickness.[22] Ginger extract at the dosage of 125 mg four times daily was shown effective in one study.[23] Traditionally, it has been used most frequently for nausea in the powdered form. Powdered ginger should be dosed at 250 g four times daily.[24,25] Two grams per day is considered a safe upper limit for consumption in pregnancy. Women must take into account the amount of ginger present in real ginger ales, in addition to their supplement.

Vitamin B_6 and doxylamine have a long history of use by midwives and physicians for nausea and vomiting in pregnancy. There are two good studies that show effectiveness of B_6 at a dose of 25 mg three times daily.[26,27] It is recommended to start with B_6, then if not totally effective, to add doxylamine at a dose of 25 mg three times daily. Patients should be warned that it may cause drowsiness.

Gastroesophageal Reflux

Reflux and heartburn are experienced frequently by pregnant women, especially as they approach term. In addition to the usual lifestyle advice, there are a few supplements that may be beneficial. Unfortunately, none have been specifically studied for treating pregnancy-related gastroesophageal reflux. Chamomile (*Matricaria recutita*) is traditionally used for dyspepsia and is safe in pregnancy.[28] It can be consumed as a tea and is noted to have sedative properties. Marshmallow root (*Althaea officinalis*) is an herb that contains mucilage polysaccharides known to coat and protect the esophagus from irritation.[29] To prepare it, patients should steep 0.5 to 1 oz of dried herb in 1 qt of hot water for 30 minutes and drink as a tea. Papaya enzyme and probiotics are also reported by the midwifery community to be helpful, but there has not been any research into their use for pregnancy-related dyspepsia.

Constipation

Constipation is prevalent among pregnant women, starting early in pregnancy and continuing into the postpartum period. Lifestyle measures, such as increasing exercise, and increasing fluid and fiber intake are a good start. Beet molasses is traditionally used at a dose of 1 to 2 tablespoons daily, and may be worth trying. Ground flaxseed, prunes, and prune juice may also be added to the diet. Magnesium supplementation at a dose of 120 mg by mouth three times daily can be titrated to stimulate one soft bowl movement daily, and is likely safe to use right up to delivery, although data are very limited.[30] Senna, aloe, and cascara sagrada are herbs commonly used for constipation, which should be avoided in pregnancy, because of the risk of dependency and possible uterine stimulating effects late in pregnancy.

LABOR PREPARATION

A lot of folklore exists in around preparation for labor. Many of these customs have never been studied. The use of evening primrose oil, red raspberry leaf tea, castor oil, and acupuncture do have some positive research behind them; however, more and better-quality studies are needed.

Evening Primrose Oil

Evening primrose oil is used widely during the last month of pregnancy by midwives in the Unites States for cervical softening. It is typically administered as two capsules intravaginally at bedtime. When used as a cervical ripening agent, it has been shown to reduce the risk of postdates presentation.[31] Five studies have been done indicating the safety of evening primrose oil, three of which were randomized controlled trials. There was one study looking at oral administration, showing that this route was not effective.[32] This is not surprising, because oral administration during pregnancy was never a traditional use. More trials assessing efficacy are needed.

Red Raspberry Leaf

Red raspberry leaf (*Rubus idaeus, R occidentalis*) has been used as uterine tonic for at least two centuries. It is purported to increase blood flow to the uterus and aid the uterine muscle fibers in more organized contraction. Many herbal texts promote its use to prevent miscarriage, prevent postdates presentation, decrease discomfort in prodromal labor, and ease morning sickness. It is commonly consumed as a tea, taken as one to three cups daily. Many studies have documented safety. There was also one recent randomized-controlled trial of 192 women that showed no adverse effects to mother or baby; shorter second stage of labor; mean difference of 10 minutes; and a lower rate of forceps use (19.3% vs 30.4%).[33]

Castor Oil

In one national survey 93% of midwives reported using castor oil to induce labor.[31] Despite this prevalence, there has been little research into the use of castor oil. Only one study looking at safety was included in a recent Cochrane review, which was small and of poor methodologic quality.[34] Outcomes that were evaluated in this study included cesarean section rate, meconium staining of amniotic fluid, and APGAR scores. All women who ingested castor oil had nausea; otherwise, outcomes were no different than for women who did not ingest castor oil. There has been no randomized-controlled trial evaluating the effectiveness of castor oil for induction of labor.

Acupuncture

A Cochrane systematic review also evaluated acupuncture for inducing labor.[35] The review identified one randomized trial, three case series, and two nonrandomized trials. The first case series used electroacupuncture at 38 to 42 weeks to successfully induce labor in 21 of 31 women. The second series, used acupuncture with and without electrical stimulation to induce labor in 10 of 12 women at 19 to 43 weeks. The third study induced labor with electroacupuncture in 78% of 41 women. The author's overall conclusion was that a well-designed randomized control trial was needed to assess clinically meaningful outcomes. Certainly, the risk of using acupuncture is low, and this may be worth trying in the patient wishing to avoid a pharmaceutical induction. Acupressure points patients can massage at home are (1) midway along the top of the trapezius muscles, if one were to draw a line from the acromion to C-7; (2) the motion sickness point at the angle between the first and second metacarpals; (3) in the semicircle around the distal medial and lateral malleoli; and (4) the little toe, all over. Massage these points for at least 2 to 3 minutes each.

Other Herbs

Many herbs have historically been used to induce labor. These include blue cohosh (*Caulophyllum thalictroides*); cotton root bark (*Gossypium herbaceum*); partridge berry (*Mitchella repens*); cramp bark (*Viburnum opulus*); and black cohosh (*Cimicifuga racemosa*). Because little to no research has been conducted on the safety of these herbs for labor induction, their use by those without training in herbal medicine is not recommended.[31]

SUPPORTING THE LABORING WOMAN
Continuous Support During Labor

"Historically, women have been attended and supported by other women during labor. However, in recent decades in hospitals worldwide, continuous support during labor has become the exception rather than the routine. Concerns about the consequent dehumanization of women's birth experiences have led to calls for a return to continuous support, by women for women, during labor."[36] To come to this conclusion, Cochrane reviewed over 16 trials of continuous support during labor, which included 13,391 women (**Box 3**). This support should include continuous presence of a birth companion who provides hands-on comfort and encouragement.

Interestingly, continuous labor support was also found to be of even greater benefit when the support provider was not a member of the hospital staff, when the support began early in labor, and when labor occurred in settings in which epidural analgesia was not routinely available.[36] In most hospitals around the country, it is the labor and delivery nurse, a member of the hospital staff, who provides support to the laboring woman. This support cannot be continuous by the very nature of hospital nursing duties. Even if each patient has their own nurse, shift change occurs, and nurses have to do increasing amounts of chart documentation, blood draws, and vital signs.

Box 3
Benefits of continuous support during labor

- Reduces the chances of having a cesarean section
- Reduces epidural or other painkiller use
- Reduces use of oxytocin (Pitocin)
- Reduces the duration of labor
- Reduces the use of forceps and vacuum extraction
- Reduces the chances of health complications and hospitalizations
- Reduces dissatisfaction with the birth experience

Data from: Hodnett ED, Gates S, Hofmeyr GJ, et al. Continuous support for women during childbirth. Cochrane Database Syst Rev 2007;3:CD003766.

Nurses are also required to keep the physician, who is almost always absent from the bedside, up-to-date with regards to the patient's progress. There are other options.

Midwifery

Certified nurse-midwives are registered nurses who have completed graduate-level training in midwifery and who have passed a national certification examination. Midwifery is legal in all 50 states and the District of Columbia. They can prescribe medication in 50 states and can practice in homes, birth centers, clinics, and hospitals. In 2006, nurse-midwives attended 11.3% of all vaginal births in the United States.[37]

The midwives model of care differs from the medical model, which physicians practice in hospital settings. The midwives model of care is based on the fact that pregnancy and birth are normal life processes. This model of care includes monitoring the physical, psychologic, and social well-being of the mother throughout the childbearing cycle; providing the mother with individualized education, counseling, and prenatal care; continuous hands-on assistance during labor and delivery; minimizing technologic interventions; and identifying and referring women who require obstetric attention.

Cochrane published a meta-analysis of 11 trials in 2008 that compared birth, neonatal, and postpartum outcomes of midwives versus physicians.[38] Midwives outperformed physicians in almost all areas. Women who delivered under the care of a midwife were more likely to have a vaginal birth, initiate breast-feeding, feel in control of their labor, and have a shorted hospital stay. These women were also less likely to use analgesia during labor, have an episiotomy, have an instrumented delivery, or experience fetal loss before 24 weeks gestation. Physicians and midwives had equal rates of fetal loss and neonatal death after 24 weeks gestation. These findings led Cochrane to conclude that all women should be offered midwifery care (**Box 4**).

A recent publication by Sakala and Corry,[39] of the nonprofit Childbirth Connection, issued collaboratively by Childbirth Connection, the Reforming States Group (a voluntary association of state-level health policymakers), and Milbank Memorial Fund, highlighted successful aspects of midwifery care. This report analyzed hundreds of the most recent studies and systematic reviews of maternity care, and emphasized the dangers of overuse of high-technologic interventions by obstetricians and the underuse of low-technologic measures to improve outcomes, which included the use of midwives and family physicians (**Box 5**).

Doulas

It is often difficult or impossible for physicians to be continuously present to support laboring women, because of the varied commitments their job entails. Acknowledging the benefits women gain from this type of support, many physicians may wish to guide their patients to a trained labor support person. A model that may be feasible for physicians is the use of a doula.

Box 4
How to find a midwife and learn more about midwifery

- American College of Nurse-Midwives, http://www.midwife.org/find.cfm
- Citizens for Midwifery, http://cfmidwifery.org/find/index.aspx
- Midwives Alliance of North America, http://mana.org/memberlist.html
- National Association of Certified Professional Midwives, http://www.nacpm.org/midwives-resources.html
- North American Registry of Midwives, http://narm.org/

> **Box 5**
> **Underuse of high-technologic, noninvasive measures**
>
> - Prenatal vitamins
> - Use of midwife or family physician
> - Continuous presence of a companion for the mother during labor
> - Upright and side-lying positions during labor and delivery, which are associated with less severe pain than lying down on one's back
> - Vaginal birth for most women who have had a previous caesarean section
> - Early mother-baby skin-to-skin contact
>
> *Data from* Sakala C, Corry M. Evidence-based maternity care: what it is and what it can achieve. Childbirth Connection and the Reforming States Group; 2008. Available at: www.childbirthconnection.org/article.asp?ok=10575#.

Doula is a Greek word meaning a "woman who serves." A birth doula is a specially trained birth companion, not a friend or loved one, who provides labor support. She performs no clinical tasks, nor does she give medical advice. She is simply present to provide hands-on support to the laboring woman (**Box 6**).

To find a Doula, one can visit the Web site of Doulas of North America, at http://www.dona.org/.

A randomized controlled trial looking at doulas was done with 420 nulliparous middle-income or upper-income women, accompanied by their male partners.[40] Women were randomized to receive either doula support during labor, or to receive the standard support of nursing staff and only their spouses. Obstetric care was provided by private obstetricians. In-line with what Cochrane has described for other types of continuous support in labor, the results of doula use were positive. The cesarean section rate was 13% in the doula group and 25% among the control group. For women undergoing induction, cesarean section rates were 13% vs 59%. The doula group also had a lower rate of epidural analgesia (65% vs 76%). There have been several other studies that have had similar results in different groups of women.

PAIN RELIEF IN LABOR

Whether or not a woman has the benefit of continuous support during labor, other non-medication approaches are available that may aid pain relief. Research is sparse for

> **Box 6**
> **What questions should patients ask when interviewing a doula?**
>
> - Is she certified?
> - What does she charge, and what is in her service package?
> - How many clients does she take per month?
> - What are her backup arrangements?
> - Does she have any limitations on where she will go or which doctors and midwives she works with?
> - Does she provide references?
> - Does she do home visits?

most nonmedication approaches. Some methods that are potentially effective include the use of warm water emersion, sterile water papules, positioning, acupuncture, self-hypnosis, and warm packs.

Waterbirth

Warm water emersion, or waterbirth, has been used to aid labor for centuries, and has recently gained in popularity in the United States. Proponents of waterbirth claim that it aids in relaxation, provides pain relief, lowers adrenalin levels, and improves blood supply to the placenta. Most of these claims have not been studied.

There has been one large prospective study of 513 patients who requested waterbirth that found that patients who labored in water used less analgesia and anesthesia during labor, had a shorter duration of first and second stages of labor, and lower perineal tears and episiotomy rate.[41] No differences were seen in APGAR scores, fetal arterial and venous pH, admission rate to NICU, or infection rate. One Cochrane review was also published on waterbirth in 2006. It concluded that more studies are needed to better assess safety and efficacy.[42]

Sterile Water Papules

The use of sterile water papules is a lesser-known technique to help reduce the pain of back labor. It involves injecting 0.1 mL of sterile water into four areas just under the skin of the lower back. This is thought to provide nerve stimulation that distracts from pain. It can provide relief for 2 to 3 hours, and can be repeated. There has been one randomized, placebo-controlled trial of 272 women, which showed effectiveness and safety.[43]

Positioning

Positioning of the laboring woman's body has long been the cornerstone of midwifery skills for facilitating delivery and also for aiding in pain management. Entire books have been written on the subject of positioning the laboring woman, but little research has been done in this area. A systematic review published in 2002 concluded that an upright position in stage I of labor aided in pain relief, and the same was found for squatting in stage II.[44] It was also concluded that squatting facilitated a faster delivery. For more information on positioning the laboring woman, *The Labor Progress Handbook* by Simkin and Ancheta is a good resource.[45]

Acupuncture and Self-hypnosis

A Cochrane review published in 2006 looked at a few selected methods of nonpharmacologic pain relief in labor.[46] The reviewers included 14 trials involving 1537 women. They concluded that women taught self-hypnosis used less pharmacologic analgesia, including epidural analgesia. The trials of acupuncture also showed a decreased need for pain relief. No objective benefit was seen for women receiving aromatherapy or audio analgesia.

Warm Packs

The use of warm packs is commonplace in most hospitals in the United States and the data on their benefit are interesting. A large randomized-controlled trial of 717 women published in 2007 showed that the application of warm packs to the perineum starting late in the second stage of labor significantly reduced the risk of third- and fourth-degree laceration.[47] Use of warm packs also reduced pain during birth and in the immediate postpartum period. Some indication also existed that warm packs may

Table 1
Evidence-based practice recommendations

Practice Recommendations	Evidence Rating	References
Pregnant women in the United States should supplement their diet with omega-3 fatty acids	A	4–10
Pregnant women should supplement their diets with vitamin D	B	12–16
Pregnant women with a strong personal or family history of atopic disease should take probiotics during the the third trimester of pregnancy	B	17,18
Acupuncture and acupressure are safe and effective for treatment of nausea and vomiting in pregnancy	B	21
Ginger is safe and effective for treatment of nausea and vomiting in pregnancy	A	22–25
Vitamin B$_6$ is safe and effective for the treatment of nausea and vomiting in pregnancy	A	26,27
Chamomile and marshmallow root are herbs that are beneficial in the treatment of gastroesophageal reflux disease in pregnancy	C	28,29
Magnesium supplementation is safe and effective for treatment of constipation in pregnancy	B	30
Evening primrose oil may be used intravaginally as a cervical ripening agent during the final weeks of pregnancy	B	31,32
Red raspberry leaf tea may be taken during pregnancy to shorten the second stage of labor and decrease the risk of forceps use	B	33
Castor oil is safe and effective when taken orally to induce labor	C	34
Acupuncture and acupressure are safe and effective for induction of labor	B	35
All laboring women should have the continuous presence of a birth companion who provides hands-on comfort and encouragement	A	36
Midwifery care of low-risk women yields superior outcomes when compared with physician care	A	38
Following the midwifery model of care, physicians should decrease the inappropriate use of high-tech interventions, and increase the use of proved low-tech interventions to improve outcomes	A	39
The use of a doula for laboring women decreases the risk of cesarean section and also decreases the use of analgesia	A	40
Warm water immersion is a safe and effective means of pain relief in labor	C	41,42
Sterile water papules are safe and effective for relief of back pain in labor	B	43
Women should be encouraged to maintain an upright position during stage I of labor and should be encouraged to squat during stage II	B	44
Self-hypnosis and acupuncture decrease the need for analgesia during labor	A	46
Warm packs should be applied to the perineum late in stage II of labor to reduce pain and decrease the risk of laceration	A	47

Level A: High-quality, randomized, double-blinded, controlled clinical trials with adequate sample size and statistical power.
Level B: Randomized trials of lesser statistical power (eg, single-blinded), cohort, and case-controlled studies.
Level C: Expert opinion or "practice pearls," which may not be rigorously substantiated through trials in the literature.

reduce the risk of urinary incontinence at 3 months postpartum, although the data for this were not as strong.

SUMMARY

There are many options for natural and preventative therapies during pregnancy and childbirth that aid in minimizing the use of pharmaceuticals and invasive procedures. Patients may seek these out, and it is important as physicians to have some basic knowledge to guide their choices. **Table 1** lists evidence-based practice recommendations. Of all therapies, the most important are nutrition for optimizing health and the provision of continuous support during labor. With the use of these measures, women in conjunction with their physicians can feel empowered to create a positive pregnancy and birth experience.

REFERENCES

1. Tsui B, Dennehy CE, Tsourounis C. A survey of dietary supplement use during pregnancy at an academic medical center. Am J Obstet Gynecol 2001;185:433.
2. Hollyer T, Boon H, Georgouis A, et al. The use of CAM by women suffering from nausea and vomiting during pregnancy. BMC Complement Altern Med 2002;2:5.
3. Glover DG, Amonkar M, Rybeck BF, et al. Prescription, over-the-counter, and herbal medicine use in a rural obstetric population. Am J Obstet Gynecol 2003;188:1039–45.
4. Benisek D, Shabert J, Skomik R. Dietary intake of polyunsaturated fatty acids by pregnant or lactating women in the United States. Obstet Gynecol 2000;95:77–8.
5. Otto SJ, Van Houwelingen AC, Antal M, et al. Maternal and neonatal essential fatty acid status in phospholipids: an international comparative study. Eur J Clin Nutr 1997;51:232–42.
6. Min Y, Ghebremeskel K, Crawford MA, et al. Pregnancy reduces arachidonic and docosahexaenoic in plamsa triacylglycerols of Korean women. Int J Vitam Nutr Res 2000;70:70–5.
7. Al MD, Van Houwelingen AC, Kester ADM, et al. Maternal essential fatty acid patterns during normal pregnancy and their relationship to the neonatal essential fatty acids status. Br J Nutr 1995;74:55–68.
8. McGregor JA, Allen KG, Harris MA, et al. The omega-3 story: nutritional prevention of preterm birth and other adverse pregnancy outcomes. Obstet Gynecol Surv 2001;56(5 Suppl 1):S1–13.
9. Carlson SE. Docosahexaenoic acid and arachidonic acid in infant development. Semin Neonatol 2001;6(5):437–49.
10. Dunstan JA, Simmer K, Dixon G, et al. Cognitive assessment of children at age 2(1/2) years after maternal fish oil supplementation in pregnancy: a randomised controlled trial. Arch Dis Child Fetal Neonatal Ed 2008;93(1):F45–50.
11. Foran SE, Flood JG, Lewandrowski KB. Measurement of mercury levels in concentrated over-the-counter fish oil preparations: is fish oil healthier than fish? Arch Pathol Lab Med 2003;127(12):1603–5.
12. Hollis BW, Horst RL. The assessment of circulating 25(OH)D and 1,25(OH)2D: where we are and where we are going. J Steroid Biochem Mol Biol 2007;103: 473–6.
13. Holick MF. Vitamin D deficiency. N Engl J Med 2007;357:266–81.
14. Hollis BW, Wagner CL, Kratz A, et al. Normal serum vitamin D levels. N Engl J Med 2005;352:515–6.

15. Wagner C, Taylor S, Hollis B. Does vitamin D make the world go round? Breast-feed Med 2008;3(4):239–50.
16. Merewood A, Mehta SD, Chen TC, et al. Association between vitamin D deficiency and primary cesarean section. J Clin Endocrinol Metab. 2009;94(3): 940–5.
17. Lee J, Seto D, Bielory L. Meta-analysis of clinical trials of probiotics for prevention and treatment of pediatric atopic dermatitis. J Allergy Clin Immunol 2008;121(1): 116–21.
18. Kuitunen M, Kukkonen K, Juntunen-Backman K, et al. Probiotics prevent IgE-associated allergy until age 5 years in cesarean-delivered children but not in the total cohort. J Allergy Clin Immunol 2009;123(2):335–41.
19. Noble E. Essential exercises for the childbearing year: a guide to health and comfort before and after your baby is born. 4th edition. Harwich: New Life Images; 2003.
20. DiGaetano A. Nausea and vomiting in pregnancy. In: Rakel D, editor. Integrative medicine. 2nd edition. Philadelphia: Saunders; 2007. p. 581–7.
21. Fugh-Berman A. Acupressure for nausea and vomiting of pregnancy. Alt Ther Women's Health 1999;1:9–16.
22. Borrelli F, Capasso R, Aviello G, et al. Effectiveness and safety of ginger in the treatment of pregnancy-induced nausea and vomiting. Obstet Gynecol 2005; 106(3):640–1.
23. Portnoi G, Chng LA, Karimi-Tabesh L, et al. Prospective comparative study of the safety and effectiveness of ginger for the treatment of nausea and vomiting in pregnancy. Am J Obstet Gynecol 2003;189:1374–7.
24. Fischer-Rasmussen W. Ginger and the treatment of hyperemesis gravidarum. Eur J Obstet Gynecol Reprod Biol 1990;38:19–24.
25. Vutyavanich T, Kraisarin T, Ruangsri R. Ginger for nausea and vomiting in preg-nancy: randomized, double-masked, placebo-controlled trial. Obstet Gynecol 2001;97:577–82.
26. Sahakian V, Rouse D, Sipes S, et al. Vitamin B6 therapy for nausea and vomiting of pregnancy: a randomized, double-blind placebo-controlled study. Obstet Gynecol 1991;78:33–6.
27. Vutyavanich T, Wongtra-ngan S, Ruangsri R. Pyridoxine for nausea and vomiting of pregnancy: a randomized, double blind, placebo-controlled trial. Am J Obstet Gynecol 1995;173:881–4.
28. Madisch A, Holtmann G, Mayr G, et al. Treatment of functional dyspepsia with a herbal preparation: a double-blind, randomized, placebo-controlled, multi-center trial. Digestion 2004;69:45–52.
29. Basch E, Ulbricht C, Hammerness P, et al. Marshmallow (Althaea officinalis L.) monograph. J Herb Pharmacother. 2003;3(3):71–81.
30. Meier B, Huch R, Zimmermann R, et al. Does continuing magnesium supplemen-tation until delivery affect labor and puerperium outcome? Eur J Obstet Gynecol Reprod Biol 2005;123(2):157–61.
31. McFarlin BL, Gibson MH, O'Rear J, et al. A national survey of herbal preparation use by nurse-midwives for labor stimulation: review of the literature and recom-mendations for practice. J Nurse Midwifery. 1999;44(6):602–3.
32. Dove D, Johnson P. Oral evening primrose oil: its effect on length of pregnancy and selected intrapartum outcomes in low risk nulliparous women. J Nurse Midwifery 1999;44:320–4.
33. Simpson M, Parsons M, Greenwood J, et al. Raspberry leaf in pregnancy: its safety and efficacy in labor. J Midwifery Womens Health 2001;46:51–9.

34. Kelly AJ, Kavanagh J, Thomas J. Castor oil, bath and/or enema for cervical priming and induction of labour. Cochrane Database Syst Rev 2001;(2):CD003099.
35. Smith CA, Crowther CA. Acupuncture for induction of labour. Cochrane Database Syst Rev 2004;(1):CD002962.
36. Hodnett ED, Gates S, Hofmeyr GJ, et al. Continuous support for women during childbirth. Cochrane Database Syst Rev 2007;(3):CD003766.
37. Martin JA, Hamilton BE, Sutton PD, et al. In: Births: final data for 2006. National vital statistics reports. Hyattsville (MD): National Center for Health Statistics; 2009;57(7):1–104.
38. Hatem M, Sandall J, Devane D, et al. Midwife-led versus other models of care for childbearing women. Cochrane Database Syst Rev 2008;(4):CD004667.
39. Sakala C, Corry M. Evidence-based maternity care: what it is and what it can achieve. Co-published with Childbirth Connection and the Reforming States Group; 2008. Available at: www.childbirthconnection.org/article.asp?ok=10575#.
40. McGrath SK, Kennell JH. A randomized controlled trial of continuous labor support for middle-class couples: effect on cesarean delivery rates. Birth 2008; 35:92–7.
41. Zanetti-Dallenbach R, Lapaire O, Maertens A, et al. Water birth, more than a trendy alternative: a prospective, observational study. Arch Gynecol Obstet 2006;274(6):355–65.
42. Cluett ER, Nikodem VC, McCandlish RE, et al. Immersion in water in pregnancy, labour and birth. Cochrane Database Syst Rev 2004;(2):CD000111.
43. Trolle B, Moller M, Kronborg H, et al. The effect of sterile water blocks on low back labor pain. Am J Obstet Gynecol 1991;164:1277–81.
44. Simkin PP, O'hara M. Nonpharmacologic relief of pain during labor: systematic reviews of five methods. Am J Obstet Gynecol 2002;186:S131–59.
45. Simkin P, Ancheta R. The labor progress handbook: early interventions to prevent and treat dystocia. 1st edition. Oxford: Blackwell Publishers; 2000.
46. Smith CA, Collins CT, Cyna AM, et al. Complementary and alternative therapies for pain management in labour. Cochrane Database Syst Rev 2006;(4): CD003521.
47. Dahlen HG, Homer CS, Cooke M, et al. Perineal outcomes and maternal comfort related to the application of perineal warm packs in the second stage of labor: a randomized controlled trial. Birth 2007;34(4):282–90.

Biofield Therapies: Energy Medicine and Primary Care

J. Adam Rindfleisch, MD, MPhil

KEYWORDS

- Integrative medicine • Biofield • Energy medicine
- Healing touch • Therapeutic touch • Reiki

Energy medicine modalities are perhaps the most mysterious and controversial of approaches used in complementary/alternative medicine (CAM). Although such practices have been an essential part of shamanic and other healing practices for as long as human communities have existed,[1] scientific investigation of energy medicine is in its early stages; much remains to be learned about mechanisms of action and efficacy.

An estimated 0.5% of Americans have used some form of energy medicine in the past year, according to the 2007 National Health Information Survey, which included 23,300 Americans.[2] A similar survey released by the Centers for Disease Control in 2004 indicated that 0.5% of participants had used qi gong and 1.0% had used reiki.[3] These numbers may in actuality be much higher than survey data indicates, given that many CAM and other providers of therapies not formally classed as energy medicine-based (eg, massage therapists, chiropractors, and herbalists) also incorporate energy medicine into their practices. At least 50 hospitals and clinics in the United States offer energy healing to patients in some form.[4]

This article defines energy medicine and outlines key elements biofield therapies have in common. Several specific approaches are described, some of which are now incorporated into allopathic clinics and hospitals. Research findings related to efficacy are summarized. Proposed mechanisms of action and safety issues are also discussed. Guidelines are offered for primary care providers wishing to advise patients about energy medicine or to integrate it into their practices, and resources for obtaining additional information are provided.

DEFINITIONS

Daniel J. Benor, a physician who has written extensively on energy medicine, defines it as follows

---

The author has no grant support to disclose.

Department of Family Medicine, Odana Atrium Family Medicine Clinic, University of Wisconsin School of Medicine and Public Health, 5618 Odana Road, Madison, WI 53719, USA

E-mail address: adam.rindfleisch@fammed.wisc.edu

The term energy medicine derives from the perceptions and beliefs of therapists and patients that there are subtle, biologic energies that surround and permeate the body. It is suggested that these energies may be accessed in various ways through CAM for diagnostic and therapeutic interventions.[5]

The energy field of the body is often referred to as the biofield, and these modalities may also be referred to as biofield therapies.

The National Center for Complementary and Alternative Medicine (NCCAM) categorizes energy medicine modalities using two main classes.[6] Modalities in the first class, veritable energy modalities, use forms of energy that are measurable using conventional technology. The second class, the putative (or subtle) energy modalities, claims to measure or manipulate forms of energy that have not been definitively, scientifically measured. Putative energy modalities, such as reiki, healing touch, and quantum touch, are the focus of this article because they are the best-studied approaches to date. For many practitioners of energy medicine, these categorizations seem arbitrary; some claim that means do in fact exist (eg, semiconducting quantum interference devices, orgone boxes, special types of galvanometers, and Kirlian photography) for measuring the subtle energy of the body.[7] Key concepts common to many biofield/ energy modalities are outlined in **Box 1**.

TYPES OF BIOFIELD/ENERGY THERAPIES

Table 1 lists modalities that are commonly classed as energy healing modalities, with brief descriptions.

MECHANISM OF ACTION

It is well known that the body emits and is influenced by energy. ECG, EEG, EMG, MRI, and numerous other diagnostic and therapeutic interventions make use of the energetic properties of the body. If two people are in close proximity, each person's EEG and EKG patterns will influence the other's.[8] Living things are known to release different quantities of light energy, or biophotons.[9] Pulsed magnetic-field therapy has been used to facilitate healing of challenging fractures for many years.[10] However, there is no single, scientifically validated theory of how putative energy modalities might work. Scientific theories about energy medicine's mechanisms of action abound; many of them hold that biofield energy lies somewhere on the electromagnetic spectrum. Many draw heavily from the findings and theories of quantum physics.

The Biofield Hypothesis

The biofield hypothesis is one explanatory model that draws from physics to conceptualize how subtle energy arises and behaves:

The biofield is defined here as the endogenous, complex dynamic electromagnetic (EM) field resulting from the superposition of component EM fields of the organism... The components of the biofield are the EM fields contributed by each individual oscillator or electrically charged, moving particle or ensembles of particles of the organism (ion, molecule, cell, tissue, and so forth), according to principles of conventional physics. The resulting biofield may be conceived of as a very complex dynamic standing wave. It has a broad spectral bandwidth, being composed of many different EM frequencies, analogous to a musical symphony with many harmonics that change over time.[11]

Biofield models attempt to account for the nonlinear, self-organizing, and dynamic qualities that define biologic systems; in a way, they attempt to characterize a more

Box 1
Key concepts common to many biofield/energy modalities

- Energy workers hold that, in addition to the physical body, an energy body exists that has a direct influence on health. Problems with the energy body can precede physical problems. Similarly, a positive change at the energetic level can lead to physical healing.

- The energy body is described in terms of its own anatomy. Different levels of energy fields (the aura) are commonly described, as are chakras, which are centers of energy whose roles vary according to their location in or around the body. Some modalities, such as acupuncture, focus on meridians, or energy channels, that course through the body.

- The energy body is in constant flux according to individuals' emotional, physical, mental, and other states. It is held that energy follows the intentions of both the healer and the person receiving the healing.

- Energy workers use a variety of techniques to perceive the energy body. Some healers profess to see energy, where others feel it by touch or hear information that guides therapy. Intuition is highly valued. Many therapists use muscle testing, in which a particular muscle group's strength is tested in response to a given question. A decrease in strength is said to indicate a negative answer. Some therapists use dowsing, in which the movement of a pendulum or other object is said to reflect the quantity or direction of energy flow.

- Many biofield therapists hold that they can maneuver the energy body through various means. Some claim to do so simply by directing their intention; others use their hands. Stones, tuning forks, colors, visualization exercises, chanting, breathing practices, and many other approaches may also be used.

- Most healers have experienced a health crisis, or healer's journey, themselves that led to their energy medicine interest and/or skills.

- Some healers begin sessions with a detailed intake form, covering the medical and other past history of the person to receive healing. Others will simply focus on where they are drawn by intuition.

- Training in various modalities varies. Some practices, such as healing touch, require years of training, with hundreds of hours of documented time with clients required for certification. Many healers describe what they do as a gift that they have cultivated without formal training.

- Often, energy healers will warn that health conditions will worsen briefly after treatment before improving.

- Energy healing can complement allopathic approaches. Many hospitals incorporate reiki, therapeutic touch, or healing touch, particularly to help people before or after surgery or cancer treatment.

- Problems may arise when patients defers biomedical interventions for an extended period of time to pursue energy modalities.

- Nonlocality (described later) is intrinsic to biofield healing. Many energy workers claim they can assist their clients without being in physical proximity to them.

- Spirituality often comes into play in energy healing sessions. Some healers claim to be assisted by non-physical beings (sometimes referred to as guides or angels) who guide the healing process. Some healers also discuss the roles played by past life experiences, reincarnation, or karma.

- In a typical healing encounter, the person receiving energy work may perceive physical sensations, such as tingling, temperature changes, pressure, or other sensory impressions. Intense emotional experiences and memories may also surface.

Data from Refs.[4,8–14]

Table 1
Energy healing modalities

Energy Modality	Description and Related Web Site[a]
Acupuncture/ acupressure	Needles are inserted into points that are said to be located along different meridians, or energy channels, within the body. In electroacupuncture, electricity is passed through the needles. In acupressure, the points are stimulated by touch. http://www.yinyanghouse.com/
Emotional freedom technique, thought field therapy	Created by Gary Craig and Roger Callahan, respectively. Tapping of various meridian points is said to release stored negative emotional energy. http://www.emofree.com/, http://www.rogercallahan.com/index.php
Polarity therapy	Based on the work of Randolph Stone. Combines diet, exercise, and other techniques to optimize the health of the energy field. http://www.polaritytherapy.org/
Reiki	Originated in Japan with Mikao Usui. Trainees are given attunements said to allow them to pass universal healing energy through them to others. Many different schools exist. http://www.reiki.com/
Therapeutic touch	Developed by Dolores Krieger, a nurse, and Dora Kunz in the 1970s. Gentle touch is used to influence the biofield. http://www.therapeutictouch.org/
Healing touch	Developed in the 1980s by Janet Mentgen, a registered nurse. Based on principles used in therapeutic touch and other such techniques. Extensive instruction and training required for certification. http://www.healingtouchinternational.org/
Quantum touch	Created by Richard Gordon. Energy is directed through intention, breath work, and other techniques. Strong focus on musculoskeletal issues, among others. http://www.quantumtouch.com/
Barbara Brennan School of Healing.	Focuses on energy healing according to detailed descriptions of energy anatomy and flow. There are many schools of healing based on the experiences/techniques of a specific individual and this is one example. http://www.barbarabrennan.com/
Flower essences	Various flower extracts are said to influence people according to the nature/energy of their plants of origin. http://www.bachcentre.com/
Eye movement desensitization and reprocessing	Rapid alternation of eye movements from left to right and tapping of specific groups of points on the body are used in various patterns to release energy-based problems. http://www.emdr.com/
Crystal therapy/gem therapy	Use of minerals to influence the energy field. Different stones are thought to have specific vibrational properties. http://healing.about.com/od/crystaltherapy/Crystal_Therapy.htm
Qi gong	Enlists various precise body movements to alter one's capacity to store and manipulate qi, or energy. http://www.qigonginstitute.org/main_page/main_page.php
Reflexology	Certain parts of the feet, believed to correlate with various body parts are massaged or treated with essential oils. http://www.reflexology-usa.org/
Shamanic healing	Often classed as a spiritual, rather than energetic, modality. The healer intuitively determines the source of a health problem and enlists ritual, helpful spirits, journeys to the spirit world, or other techniques to bring about healing. http://www.shamanresource.com/

[a] Although some of the Web sites listed do include some research data, they are provided primarily as a way for readers to familiarize themselves with various modalities in greater detail. This list is by no means comprehensive. Many complementary/alternative medicine therapies can be considered to be energy-based in part. Medical systems, such as Ayurveda, Traditional Chinese Medicine, and homeopathy incorporate energy medicine in various ways. Many schools of yoga and meditation also involve energy awareness and manipulation.

sophisticated form of the homeostasis seen at a cellular level. The biofield hypothesis posits that the complex interplay of events on a small scale causes emergent properties (characteristics of a living organism, such as consciousness, relationships with others, the creation of meaning, and one's overall state of health) to arise.

Nonlocality and Entanglement

Central to many putative energy modalities is the idea that energy can be manipulated through various means. Many traditions teach that this can even occur without direct contact between a healer and the person receiving healing. *Non-locality* is a term used to describe interactions between two entities that do not depend on spatial proximity. *Entanglement* is a physics term used to describe a connection between two particles that somehow exists even though the particles are separated across space. Entanglement was first noted in a 1982 experiment by Aspect.[12] It was found that two electrons that were initially in contact with one another would continue to influence one another once separated. Changing the spin of one electron would spontaneously lead to a change in the spin of another, even though they were separated by great distances.

Human research that focuses on these principles, although controversial, bears mentioning. A 1994 study featured in *Physics Essays* suggested that human interactions may lead to a form of entanglement or connection.[13] Seven pairs of subjects were tested in two different scenarios. For the first part of the experiment, the subjects were not allowed to meet each other. Subjects were asked to relax in chairs in Faraday chambers, electromagnetically isolated rooms, that were 14.5 m apart. One subject was shown a series of 100 randomly timed flashing lights, and during the flashes, both subjects' electroencephalogram (EEG) tracings were taken. As might be expected, there was no correlation between EEG signals in response to the flashing lights.

However, this changed for some pairs of subjects in the second part of the experiment. For this phase of the experiment, the two test subjects were given time to meet one another. This included 20 minutes to "get to know one another in meditative silence." It was found that if the subjects spent time together and if they both felt they had good rapport (this occurred in two of seven pairs), they seemed to establish and maintain a nonlocal connection to one another. As one subject watched the 100 random flashing lights in the shielded chamber, their partner, 14.5 m away, also had an EEG response in the occipital cortex over the first several milliseconds of light exposure. For the first 72 milliseconds after exposure, the p value was 0.005, and at 132 milliseconds, it was 0.009. The authors concluded that it was possible for nonlocal interactions to occur between two human brains.

The methodology for the 1994 study has been challenged, but findings have been replicated elsewhere. In 2004, Radin followed the EEG results of 13 pairs of subjects after they had been asked to "maintain a feeling of connectedness" with one another for a period of time. Three of the pairs had EEG correlations that were statistically significant.[14]

Another study, conducted in Hawaii, raises the possibility that energy healing can have nonlocal effects. Eleven healers, from a variety of traditions, who claimed they could connect with or heal others from a distance, were asked to select a person with whom they felt a "strong connection." Recipients were placed in a functional MRI scanner and then the healers were asked to send "distant intentionality" to them at random 2-minute intervals. The recipients were not aware of when this was to happen. The p value for differences in MRI findings for the "send" and "no send" periods was 0.000127. It was noted that intention on the part of the healer activated the recipients' brains at the anterior and middle cingulate, precuneus, and frontal areas.[15]

Biofield Awareness

In considering claims made by energy medicine providers, one must ask not only whether or not the biofield exists but if it is possible for people to detect it. Study findings are mixed, but many suggest it is possible. A 2005 study had 165 undergraduates complete a battery of six biofield awareness tasks. These included having experimenters place their hands near a subject and evaluating awareness of the hands' proximity, detecting being stared at, and predicting others' intentions. Overall accuracy was 10.3% above chance. Subjects' sensitivity correlated with survey measures of self awareness and sensitivity to others, although most subjects underestimated how they would perform.[16] It has been noted, in the brain and in other organs, such as the heart, that the autonomic nervous system exhibits a response before certain randomly presented emotional stimuli are sensed.[17] How this might related to human healing remains to be explored.

Table 2 summarizes some proposed mechanisms of action for energy medicine modalities.

ENERGY MEDICINE'S EFFICACY: THE STATE OF THE RESEARCH

Most reviews of the most commonly researched energy therapies conclude that, although research findings show that such interventions are promising more research is needed. For example, a 2007 review concluded that studies of therapeutic touch, healing touch, and reiki are quite promising; however, at this point, they can only suggest that these healing modalities have efficacy in reducing anxiety; improving muscle relaxation; aiding in stress reduction, relaxation, and sense of well-being; promoting wound healing; and reducing pain.[29]

Research in energy medicine is gaining momentum, and increasing numbers of good-quality studies are emerging. The National Institutes of Health National Center for Complementary Alternative Medicine has funded the Center for Frontier Medicine in Biofield Science at the University of Arizona in Tucson.[30] Standards for performing biofield research have been outlined.[31] As with many modalities for which research is limited, the potential role of energy modalities within Western health care remains hotly debated.

GENERAL REVIEWS

A 2003 publication by Benor and Crawford evaluated 2200 published reports on energy medicine, spiritual healing, distant healing and prayer, concluding that most studies had weak designs, but the results indicated that further study with sounder methodologies were warranted.[32] In a summary of their findings, they stated that there is evidence, though not conclusive, to suggest an interaction between mind and matter consistent with the claims of many energy healing modalities. They suggested that, based on their review of that data, effects of intention on nonliving systems are small (<1%) but skin conductance and the autonomic nervous systems of living organisms are more strongly affected. In general, the reviewers suggested that effects of various forms of spiritual and energy healing are likely smaller than reported in the literature at the time (2003). The need for more, higher-quality research was emphasized.[33]

A systematic review of distant healing, published in 2000, included 23 trials that met inclusion criteria. Reviewers found a positive treatment effect in 13 of the trials, which

Table 2
Proposed mechanisms of action for putative energy medicine modalities[a]

Mechanism	Comment
Healing alters the body's electromagnetic field.	Magnetometers known as SQUIDs (superconducting quantum interference devices), although controversial, are said to measure large frequency biomagnetic fields radiating from therapeutic touch providers.[18] Practitioners of yoga and qi gong seem to be able to radiate fields 1000 times stronger than average, in a frequency range that has also been linked to speeding healing of biologic tissues.[19]
Energy healing alters gamma wave release, particularly by potassium-40, the body's main gamma-wave source.	Studies indicate an increase in gamma release during healing sessions.[6,7,20]
Energy healing influences the release of biophotons.[21]	It is known that biophoton release increases in stressed cells; it is correlated with oxidative stress.[22] Long-term practitioners of transcendental meditation have been noted to have much lower levels of biophoton emission than controls[23] Biophotons are thought to contribute energy to electron clouds surrounding the atoms in blood.[24]
Energy work decreases entropy.	A 2003 study hypothesized that healing intention might lead to alterations in entropy, measured as the number of times that a random event generator (REG) produced more organized patterns than would be expected by chance alone. An REG placed in a healer's office had significantly more ordered patterns than one placed in a library, when all other variables were controlled. This pattern proved true for three separate 3-month studies.[25]
Healers help patients entrain with the magnetic field of the earth.	The earth's Schumann resonance and a brain in an alpha wave pattern cycle at roughly 7–10 Hz.[26]
Energy medicine arises through the transmission of signals through a living matrix of connective tissues, including the perineurium and myofascial tissue.	The myofascial and other tissues have properties similar to crystals and function as semiconductors. Piezoelectricity, which arises when semiconducting crystalline lattices are moved in some way, may transmit energy. This is also thought to be true at the cellular level, with signal transfer that can occur throughout the body via cellular microtubules.[7,27,28]
The vibration of the healer entrains with the recipient of healing and favorably alters the recipient's energetic state.	There is evidence to show that EEG synchrony between bioenergy practitioners and clients occurs during healing.[8] One theory proposed by Oschman suggests that during meditation or other mindful states, molecules vibrating throughout the body will entrain or harmonize, creating more balanced (healthier) frequencies.[28]

[a] This list is just a small sampling of popular theories. Other mechanisms have been proposed, including alterations in electron-excited states, quantum coherence, and the ability of biologic systems to function as lasers.

Data from Oschman J. Energy medicine in therapeutics and human performance. Edinburgh: Butterworth Heinemann; 2003.

involved a total of 2774 subjects.[34] A 2003 follow-up incorporating additional studies concluded that "Collectively they shift the weight of the evidence against the notion that distant healing is more than a placebo."[35] Study findings continue to be hotly debated several years later.

Other reviews have been mixed. A 2000 review of 37 trials, 22 of which were accessible as published reports, found that 10 of them showed a significant effect. The studies varied greatly in intervention, outcomes measures, and study length. Methodological shortcomings were common, and it was concluded that no firm conclusions could be drawn based on the randomized controlled trials featured in the study.[36] Similarly, a series of meta-analyses published in 2003 indicated that most of the studies were of poor quality, although many studies had significant effect sizes.[37]

A 2008 Cochrane review of touch therapies for pain evaluated five healing touch, 16 therapeutic touch, and five reiki trials that met criteria. The total number of subjects in these studies was 1153. Pain was reduced an average of 0.83 points on a 10-point rating scale (95% CI -1.16 to -0.5). There was a significant decrease in two out of five studies that evaluated analgesic use. No significant placebo effect was found. The review concluded that "touch therapies may have a modest effect on pain relief."[38]

RESEARCH FOCUSING ON SPECIFIC MODALITIES

Therapeutic touch (TT), reiki, and healing touch (HT) are perhaps the most commonly used energy medicine therapies in the United States. These therapies, often referred to together as touch therapies, have been the focus of several studies. Qi gong has also been gaining popularity in the United States.

Therapeutic Touch

As noted earlier, therapeutic touch trials have been reviewed en masse with other energy medicine studies, but individual meta-analyses specifically related to TT are less common. A 2008 review that looked at other modalities also concluded that TT "...does help reduce pain and anxiety,"[39] but a Cochrane review found an insufficient number of studies to allow conclusions to be drawn about whether or not TT was beneficial for anxiety.[40] A 2003 Cochrane review did not find TT to be helpful in healing acute wounds.[41]

A few positive findings exist. One 2005 study did indicate that two 5- to 7-minute sessions a day of TT proved helpful for certain behaviors (vocalizations and repetitive hand movements) in subjects who had dementia.[42] A 1999 meta-analysis of 13 studies (with numerous methodological problems) noted the average study effect size for TT in a variety of scenarios was 0.39, which was described as moderate.[43]

Perhaps no research in energy medicine has generated more controversy than the Rosa Therapeutic Touch Study.[44] This 1998 study, featured in the *Journal of the American Medical Association*, documented the findings of a fourth-grade science project that set out to explore whether TT practitioners could sense the presence of another person's energy field. Twenty-one TT providers were tested by being asked to lay their hands on a table. The experimenter sat opposite the subjects behind a screen, and based on a coin toss, placed a hand 8 to 10 cm over the healer's left or right hand. Healers were asked to identify which of their hands was in proximity to the experimenter's. For 280 trials, there were 123 correct responses, with a success rate of 44%. The study concluded that, "Twenty-one experienced TT practitioners were unable to detect the investigator's energy field. Their failure to substantiate TT most fundamental claim is unrefuted evidence that the claims of TT are groundless and that further professional use is unjustified."

The study's conclusions have been subject to a great deal of discussion and debate. Some arguments against its conclusions include

- Statistical analysis was not accurate.[45]
- Lack of understanding of mechanism of action does not equate to lack of efficacy.
- Experimenter beliefs have been found to influence the outcomes of such studies.[46]
- Some research indicates that therapies are much less likely to be effective if the person receiving energy is either skeptical or in a negative state of mind.
- The study focused on sensitivity to the presence of one person by a small group of healers; generalizability is not clear.
- The study did not actually gauge healing ability per se.

Regardless of one's interpretation of the study's findings, the debate it generated speaks to the level of controversy that surrounds biofield therapies.

Reiki

Reiki is one of the most popular biofield modalities in the United States and it is used in several hospital and community programs.[47] It has been subject to several systematic reviews, most of which are unable to draw conclusions about efficacy. Lee and colleagues,[48] reviewed all reiki study data through November 2007 and identified 205 relevant studies, of which nine randomized clinical trials (RCT) met inclusion criteria. The review concluded that trial data are scarce for any one condition, with a lack of independent replications. Methodological flaws were common. Ultimately, it was concluded that "...the value of reiki remains unproven."

Vitale conducted a 2007 review that divided reiki studies into categories, with the following conclusions[49]

- Stress/relaxation and depression: one significant and three nonsignifcant findings.
- Wound healing: only one nonsignifcant study noted.
- Pain: one study with significant findings for acute pain; for chronic pain one study showed significant benefit and two studies did not.
- Change in biologic correlates: studies involving autonomic nervous system measurements are weak, as are those exploring reiki effects on hemoglobin. (A recent rat study indicated that reiki can improve heart rate homeostasis.)[50]

A recent study on reiki and fibromyalgia also did not find reiki to be of benefit.[51]

Healing Touch

As of 2002, there were over 67,000 HT providers in the United States.[52] Healing Touch International[53] routinely publishes a research survey and also makes research summaries available online.[54]

A 2004 review concluded that, although there were no generalizable results from more than 30 available studies of HT, the therapy holds promise.[55] Some studies subsequent to the review are worth noting. A 2004 evaluation of the effects of HT on indicators of well-being for 78 women who had gynecologic cancers and were undergoing radiation therapy found statistically significant improvements in vitality, pain, and physical functioning in the HT group compared with controls.[56] Another randomized clinical trial indicated that anxiety scores and length of stay were decreased in 237 hospitalized study subjects randomized to three groups when

---

Box 2
Guidelines for advising patients about energy medicine or making a referral

- Become generally familiar with the forms of energy medicine your patients are most likely to use, so that you can converse with them about their experiences. In addition to the modality-specific Web sites listed in **Table 1**, some other generally useful Web resources to consider include

  - Alternative Medicine Foundation resource guide on energy work http://amfoundation.org/energywork.htm
  - Association for the Scientific Study of Consciousness http://assc.caltech.edu/
  - British Psychological Society http://www.warwick.ac.uk/cep
  - Committee for the Scientific Investigation of Claims of the Paranormal http://www.csicop.org/
  - http://www.princeton.edu/_rdnelson/gcpintro.html
  - Institute of Noetic Sciences http://www.noetic.org/
  - International Society for the Study of Subtle Energies and Energy Medicine http://www.issseem.org/
  - Society for the Anthropology of Consciousness http://sunny.moorpark.cc.ca.us/_jbaker/sac/home.html
  - Princeton Engineering Anomalies Research http://www.princeton.edu/_pear/index.html
  - Samueli Institute for Information Biology http://www.siib.org

- Take time to meet biofield therapists in your community. Consider experiencing a session yourself.
- Evaluate healers' qualifications.

  - How much time have they spent in training?
  - Are they licensed or certified?
  - How is their knowledge of biomedicine? Providers of therapeutic touch, healing touch, and other modalities often have extensive backgrounds in nursing or other health care fields and know a great deal about anatomy, physiology, and pathology.

- Establish a dialog with a healer about shared patients, with patients' permission. Do they keep written records and are they willing to share them?
- Energy medicine is quite safe and can be considered for most complaints, but use caution in patients who have significant psychiatric disorders. Consider energy medicine when

  - A biomedical diagnostic workup has not been revealing.
  - Symptoms seem unrelated, vague, or in flux.
  - Patients make it clear that such an approach would resonate with their belief systems.

Based in part on information *from* Rakel D, Rindfleisch J. Integrative medicine. In: Rakel RE, editor. Essential of family medicine. 3rd edition. Philadelphia: Elsevier; 2006. p. 132–41.

---

they were assigned to the HT group. However, there was not a significant decrease in pain medication, antiemetic use, or atrial fibrillation incidence.[57]

Qi Gong

A few reviews have indicated a benefit from qi gong. A 2007 review on qi gong for pain conditions found that "All RCTs of external qi gong demonstrated greater pain

Table 3
Patient-oriented practice recommendations[a]

Recommendation/Conclusion	Evidence Rating	References
Energy medicine modalities can be useful when integrated with primary care medicine	C	DiNucci[4] Benor[5] Jonas & Crawford[33] Myss [60]
Biofield therapies share many common principles and assumptions	C	DiNucci[4] Myss[60] Rakel & Rindfleisch[61] Mentgen [62]Brennan [63] Feinstein et al [64] Bruyere [65] Warber et al[66]
Energy medicine is safe.	C	DiNucci[4] Benor[5,6] Jonas & Crawford[32] Myss[60] Mentgen[62] Brennan[63] Feinstein et al[64] Bruyere[65] Warber et al[66]
Nonlocal connections can be formed between pairs of people	B	Zylberbaum et al[13] Radin[14]
Healers can influence, at a distance, the fMRI readings of people with whom they feel a close connection	B	Achlerberg et al[15]
Some people seem to be aware of a biofield around themselves and others	B	Nelson & Schwartz[16]
Energy medicine modalities can influence skin conductance and autonomic function, but are less likely to affect inanimate systems	A	Jonas & Crawford[33]
Distant healing is more than just the placebo effect	B	Ernst[35]
Touch therapies modestly decrease pain (roughly 1 point on the 10-point scale)	A	So et al[38]
Therapeutic touch helps reduce pain and anxiety	C	Jackson et al[39]
Therapeutic touch does not heal acute wounds	A	O'Mathuna & Ashford[41]
Therapeutic touch may decrease some behavioral symptoms in dementia patients	B	Woods et al[42]
Healing touch improves wellbeing measures for women with gynecologic cancers undergoing radiation therapy	A	Cook et al[56]
Healing touch decreases anxiety scores in hospitalized cardiac patients, but not pain, anti-emetic use, or atrial fibrillation	A	MacIntyre et al[57]
Qigong decreases chronic pain	B	Lee et al[58]

[a] Based on the current state of the research, it is difficult to draw conclusions about the efficacy of biofield therapies for most health conditions. Different studies have conflicting results and methodological problems are common.

reductions in the qigong groups compared with control groups. Meta-analysis of two RCTs showed a significant effect of external qigong compared with general care for treating chronic pain."[58] Another review of qi gong for use in cancer care found trials that met inclusion criteria had variable methodological quality, and all of them focused on palliative/supportive care, not curative treatment. Two trials suggest that life might be prolonged, but research quality was not sufficient to support a definitive conclusion.[59]

ADVERSE EFFECTS

In general, biofield/energy modalities are thought to be quite safe. There are no reports of these interventions leading to morbidity or mortality of any duration.[4] It is not uncommon for intense emotions to arise during sessions, and many providers suggest biofield therapies should be used with caution in people who have psychoses. Patients may feel quite fatigued or dizzy after a session and many practitioners note that symptoms can momentarily worsen before they begin to improve. Recipients of energy healing often find themselves needing to confront difficult past experiences. Perhaps the most dangerous aspect of energy medicine is that there have been reports of poor outcomes when it is relied on in acute, life-threatening situations for which allopathic interventions would have a greater likelihood of decreasing morbidity and mortality.

ENERGY MEDICINE MODALITIES AND PRIMARY CARE

Box 2 outlines guidelines for practitioners advising their patients regarding the use of energy medicine modalities. Table 3 lists patient-oriented practice recommendations.

ACKNOWLEDGMENTS

Kirsten Rindfleisch, Judy Rindfleisch, Kris Helgeson, Sharon Jensen, and Mario Salguero.

REFERENCES

1. Walsh R. The World of Shamanism: new views of and ancient traditions. Woodsbury (MN): Llewelyn; 2007.
2. Barnes PM, Bloom B. Complementary and alternative medicine use among adults and children: United States, 2007. National Health Statistics Reports 2008;12. Available at: http://nccam.nih.gov/news/2008/nhsr12.pdf. Accessed August 20, 2009.
3. Barnes P, Powell-Griner E, McFann K, et al. Complementary and alternative medicine use among adults: United States, 2002. Semin Integr Med 2004;2(2):54–71.
4. DiNucci EM. Energy healing: a complementary treatment for orthopaedic and other conditions. Orthop Nurs 2005;24(4):259–69.
5. Benor DJ. Energy medicine for the internist. Med Clin North Am 2002;86(1): 105–25.
6. Energy medicine: an overview. Available at: http://nccam.nih.gov/health/what iscam/energy/energymed.htm. Accessed August 20, 2009.
7. Oschman JL. Energy medicine: the scientific basis. New York: Churchill Livingstone; 2002.
8. Russek L, Schwartz G. Energy cardiology: a dynamical energy systems approach for integrating conventional and alternative medicine. Adv Mind Body Med 1996;12(4):4–24.

9. Creath K, Schwartz GE. Biophoton images of plants: revealing the light within. J Altern Complement Med 2004;10(1):23–6.
10. Bassett CA, Mitchel SN, Gaston SR. Pulsing electromagnetic field treatment in ununited fractures and failed arthrodeses. JAMA 1982;247:623–8.
11. Rubik B. The biofield hypothesis: its biophysical basis and role in medicine. J Altern Complement Med 2002;8(6):703–7.
12. Aspect A, Dalibard J, Roger S. Experimental test of Bell's inequalities using time-varying analysers. Phy Rev Lett 1982;49:1804–7.
13. Zylberbaum JG, Delaflor M, Attie L, et al. The Einstein-Podolsky-Rosen paradox in the brain: the transferred potential. Phys Essays 1994;7(4):422–8.
14. Radin D. Event-related electroencephalographic correlations between isolated human subjects. J Altern Complement Med 2004;10:315–23.
15. Achterberg J, Cooke K, Richards T, et al. Evidence for correlations between distant intentionality and brain function in recipients: a functional magnetic resonance imaging analysis. J Altern Complement Med 2005;11(6):965–71.
16. Nelson LA, Schwartz GE. Human biofield and intention detection: individual differences. J Altern Complement Med 2005;11(1):93–101.
17. McCraty R, Atkinson M, Bradley RT. Electrophysiological evidence of intuition: part 2. A system-wide process? J Altern Complement Med 2004;10(2):325–36.
18. Zimmerman J. Laying-on-of-hands healing and therapeutic touch: a testable theory. BMEI currents. J BioElectroMagnetics Institute 1990;2:8–17.
19. Sisken BF, Walder J. Therapeutic aspects of electromagnetic fields for soft tissue healing. In: Blank M, editor. Electromagnetic fields: biological interactions and mechanisms. Washington, DC: American Chemical Society; 1995. p. 277–85.
20. Benford MS. Radiogenic metabolism: an alternative cellular energy source. Med Hypotheses 2001;56(1):33–9.
21. Choi C, Woo WM, Lee MB, et al. Biophoton emission from the hands. J Korean Phys Soc 2002;41(2):275–8.
22. Van Wijk R, Tilbury RN, Slawinski J, et al. Biophoton emission, stress and disease: a multi-author review. Experientia 1992;48:1029–102.
23. van Wijk EP, Koch H, Bosman S, et al. Anatomic characterization of human ultra-weak photon emission in practitioners of transcendental meditation and control subjects. J Altern Complement Med 2006;12(1):31–8.
24. Curtis BD, Hurtak JJ. Consciousness and quantum information processing: uncovering the foundation for a medicine of light. J Altern Complement Med 2004;10(1):27–39.
25. Crawford C, Jonas W, Nelson R, et al. Alterations in random event measures associated with a healing practice. J Altern Complement Med 2003;2(3):345–53.
26. Sentman DD. Schumann resonances. In: Volland H, editor, Handbook of atmospheric electrodynamics, vol. 1. Boca Raton (FL): CRC Press; 1995. p. 267–95.
27. Oschman J. Energy medicine in therapeutics and human performance. Edinburgh: Butterworth Heinemann; 2003.
28. Oschman JL. Clinical aspects of biological fields: an introduction for health care professionals. J Bodyw Mov Ther 2002;6(2):117–25.
29. Engebretson J, Wardell DW. Energy-based modalities. Nurs Clin North Am 2007;42(2):243–59.
30. Center for Frontier Medicine in Biofield Science. University of Arizona in Tucson. Available at: http://www.biofield.arizona.edu/CFMBS. Accessed August 20, 2009.
31. Jonas WB, Chez RA. Recommendations regarding definitions and standards in healing research. J Altern Complement Med 2004;10(1):171–81.

32. Jonas WB, Crawford CC, editors. Healing, intention and energy medicine: science, research methods, and clinical implications. New York: Churchill Livingstone; 2003.

33. Jonas WB, Crawford C. Science and spiritual healing: a critical review of spiritual healing, "energy medicine," and intentionality. Altern Ther Health Med 2003;9(2): 56–61.

34. Astin JA, Harkness E, Ernst E. The efficacy of "Distant Healing": a systematic review of randomized trials. Ann Intern Med 2000;132(11):903–10.

35. Ernst E. Distant healing–an "update" of a systematic review. Wien Klin Wochenschr 2003;115(7–8):241–5.

36. Abbot N. Healing as a therapy for human disease: a systematic review. J Altern Complement Med 2000;6(2):159–69.

37. Jonas WB, Crawford CC. Science and spiritual healing: a critical review of spiritual healing, "energy" medicine, and intentionality. Altern Ther Health Med 2003; 9(2):A56–71.

38. So PS, Jiang Y, Qin Y. Touch therapies for pain relief in adults. Cochrane Database Syst Rev 2008;(4):CD006535.

39. Jackson E, Kelley M, McNeil P, et al. Does therapeutic touch help reduce pain and anxiety in patients with cancer? Clin J Oncol Nurs 2008;12(1):113–20.

40. Robinson J, Biley FC, Dokk H. Therapeutic touch for anxiety disorders. Cochrane Database Syst Rev 2007;(3):CD006240.

41. O'Mathuna DP, Ashford RL. Therapeutic touch for healing acute wounds. Cochrane Database Syst Rev 2003;(4):CD002766.

42. Woods DL, Craven RF, Whitney J. The effect of therapeutic touch on behavioral symptoms of persons with dementia. Altern Ther Health Med 2005;11:66–74.

43. Winstead-Fry P, Kijek J. An integrative review and meta-analysis of therapeutic touch research. Altern Ther Health Med 1999;5(6):58–67.

44. Rosa L, Rosa E, Sarner L, Barrett S. A close look at therapeutic touch. JAMA 1998;279:1005–10.

45. Cox T. Applying skeptical thinking to Emily Rosa's therapeutic touch study: a nurse-statistician reanalyzes the data. Altern Ther Health Med 2002;9(1):58–64.

46. Dossey L. Therapeutic touch at the crossroads: observations on the Rosa study. Altern Ther Health Med 2003;9(1):38–9.

47. Miles P, True G. Reiki- Review of a biofield therapy: history, theory, practice, and research. Altern Ther Health Med 2003;9(2):62–72.

48. Lee MS, Pittler MH, Ernst E. Effects of Reiki in clinical practice: a systematic review of randomised clinical trials. Int J Clin Pract 2008;62(6):947–54.

49. Vitale A. An integrative review of Reiki touch therapy research. Holist Nurs Pract 2007;21(4):167–79.

50. Baldwin AL, Wagers C, Schwartz GE. Reiki improves heart rate homeostasis in laboratory rats. J Altern Complement Med 2008;14(4):417–22.

51. Assefi N, Bogard A, Goldberg J, et al. Reiki for the treatment of fibromyalgia: a randomized controlled trial. J Altern Complement Med 2008;14(9):1115–22.

52. Mentgen JL. Healing touch class news. Healing Touch Newsletter 2002;2(1):6.

53. Healing touch international. Available at: http://www.HealingTouchInternational. org. Accessed August 20, 2009.

54. Wardell DW. Healing touch research survey. 9th edition. Houston (TX): Healing Touch International; 2008.

55. Wardell DW, Weymouth KF. Review of studies of healing touch. J Nurs Scholarsh 2004;36(2):147–54.

56. Cook CA, Guerrerio JF, Slater VE. Healing touch and quality of life in women receiving radiation treatment for cancer: a randomized controlled trial. Altern Ther Health Med 2004;10(3):34–40.

57. MacIntyre B, Hamilton J, Fricke T, et al. The efficacy of healing touch in coronary artery bypass surgery recovery: a randomized clinical trial. Altern Ther Health Med 2008;4(4):24–32.

58. Lee MS, Pittler MH, Ernst E. External qigong for pain conditions: a systematic review of randomized clinical trials. J Pain 2007;8(11):827–31.

59. Lee MS, Chen KW, Sancier KM, et al. Qigong for cancer treatment: a systematic review of controlled clinical trials. Acta Oncol 2007;46(6):717–22.

60. Myss CM. Anatomy of the spirit. The seven stages of power and healing. New York: Random House; 1996.

61. Rakel D, Rindfleisch J. Integrative Medicine. In: Rakel RE, editor. Essential of family medicine. 3rd edition. Philadelphia: Elsevier; 2006. p. 132–41.

62. Mentgen JL. Healing touch. Nurs Clin North Am 2001;36(1):143–58.

63. Brennan BA. Hands of light: a guide to healing through the human energy field. New York: Bantam Dell; 1993.

64. Feinstein D, Eden D. Six pillars of energy medicine: clinical strengths of a complementary paradigm. Altern Ther Health Med 2008;14(1):44–54.

65. Bruyere RL. Wheels of light: chakras, auras, and the healing energy of the body. New York: Fireside; 1994.

66. Warber C, Deogracia C, Straughn J, et al. Biofield energy healing from inside. J Altern Complement Med 2004;10(6):1107–13.

Integrative Primary Care and the Internet: Opportunities and Challenges

Marsha J. Handel, MLS

KEYWORDS

- Internet • Integrative medicine • Complementary therapies
- Medical informatics • Information dissemination

The Internet: gateway to reliable clinical and research information or floodgate to unsubstantiated information of insufficient depth and variable quality? Can it help the physician locate high-quality information that will enhance patient care? Can it help patients become more knowledgeable, involved, and competent in participating in their health care management? Can it be used efficiently and effectively during a busy practice day to immediately educate providers and patients right at point of care? The answer to all these questions is yes. This article will empower readers with knowledge of authoritative Web sites that directly addresses clinical questions, are easy to search, and will help physicians guide their patients to sources of information that are valid and trustworthy.

Widespread use of the Internet for medical information is a relatively new phenomenon. The National Library of Medicine (NLM) only began offering public access to Medline (PubMed) in 1997. As physicians and consumers increasingly rely on the Internet for health information, the level of quality and authority continues to concern the medical informatics community. Although review mechanisms to certify reliability have been developed by organizations such as HonCode (using voluntary standards) and URAC (using independent verification), a robust discussion continues on their value for both Web publishers and end users, and new strategies for Web evaluation continue to be developed.[1–4]

The issue of information quality in integrative medicine is particularly cogent. Much of this information previously was driven by commercial and personal sites, providing little use to the physician and often unverified information to the consumer. Over the last 10 years, this situation has changed significantly. Research on integrative medicine has increased exponentially, and its study and practice have been adopted by

Informatics and Online Education, Department of Integrative Medicine, Beth Israel Medical Center, 245 Fifth Avenue, New York, NY 10016, USA
E-mail address: mhandel@chpnet.org

Prim Care Clin Office Pract 37 (2010) 181–200
doi:10.1016/j.pop.2009.09.006
0095-4543/10/$ – see front matter © 2010 Elsevier Inc. All rights reserved.

major academic institutions and government entities. This is evidenced by such developments as

The growth of the National Center for Complementary and Alternative Medicine (NCCAM), now a National Institutes of Health (NIH) institute supporting research and education in integrative approaches

The development of a separate subset of Medline by the NLM (the complementary and alternative medicine [CAM] database)

The formation of the Consortium of Academic Health Centers for Integrative Medicine (CACHIM), a consortium of 44 major academic medical centers in the United States and Canada

The recent Institute of Medicine *Summit on Integrative Medicine and the Health of the Public* on the role of integrative health care in light of the current US health care crisis.

Both physicians and consumers now can access an increasing amount of evidence-based information on integrative approaches to health conditions produced by reliable sources including professional organizations, government agencies, and academic institutions. This information is available through Web sites, medical and specialized databases, and evidence-based medicine (EBM) sites.

INFORMATION INTERESTS OF PHYSICIANS AND PATIENTS

Physicians increasingly have come to rely on the Internet for their professional development and clinical and research needs. Physicians rate source credibility, relevance, unlimited access, speed, and ease of use as the most important aspects of successful Internet use.[5,6]

Although physician comfort level and expertise in using the Internet have grown, searching for reliable information on integrative approaches is another issue. A study at the University Of California, San Francisco showed that physicians are frequently unable to locate the integrative information they need (most often on herbal medicine, relaxation exercises, and acupuncture), and most have little knowledge of existing authoritative resources in the field. About half the respondents rated their integrative searches as being only partially successful, and as a result, most relied on Medline searching for their information needs in this area.[7]

The 2006 Pew Survey has provided a good deal of information on consumer search behavior. It confirmed that 75% of Americans now use the Internet for health information and have a high level of interest in integrative medical topics. In fact, the top nine issues researched included specific medical conditions or treatments, diet/nutrition/supplements, mental health issues, exercise, alternative or complementary approaches, and social/emotional support. Unfortunately, the survey also revealed that 75% of health seekers do not consistently check the source and date of the health information they find online. This is of concern, because 53% of online health seekers report their most recent search affected a decision about how to treat an illness, changed their overall approach to maintaining their health or the health of another, or led them to ask a doctor new questions or get a second opinion from another doctor.[8] A literature review also revealed that Internet searches are done by the patient before a clinical encounter to determine if professional help is necessary and after a clinical encounter for reassurance or because of dissatisfaction with the amount of detailed information provided by the health professional during the visit.[9]

Another robust consumer trend is the use of disease-specific online communities and Web sites run by patients with particular health conditions. Within these forums, discussion of integrative approaches is most common for diseases in which conventional care has the least to offer or in which there is dissatisfaction with the conventional treatment approach. Although physicians may fear the accuracy of information posted on these sites, support group communities actually have been found to be impressively expert places, with misleading information consistently challenged and corrected.[10] Examples of high-quality moderated websites include

http://www.diabetes.org, the message board of the American Diabetes Association

http://my.americanheart.org/jiveforum/index.jspa for stroke survivors and family caregivers

http://www.addictionrecoryguide.com for people dealing with drug and alcohol addiction

http://apps.komen.org/Forums/, the world's largest grassroots network of breast cancer survivors and activists.

PHYSICIAN–PATIENT RELATIONSHIP

A recent government study cited that 38.3% of US adults use integrative medicine and CAM, a number that has been stable for the last 10 years.[11] Surveys show patients not only are using integrative approaches, but want increasing access to this type of information.[12,13] This level of interest and use has impacted the physician–patient relationship. Physicians are responding to the more Internet-informed patient in several ways:

Maintaining a physician-centered relationship based on the physician's expert opinion, ignoring the online information the patient has found

Cultivating a patient-centered relationship where the physician and patient collaborate in obtaining and analyzing the information

Assuming the role of physician as educator, helping patients locate reliable health information on the Internet.[9]

BARRIERS TO EFFECTIVE SEARCHING

Although both groups increasingly rely on the Internet, there are still significant barriers to satisfactory searching, primarily finding the appropriate level of information, in a reasonable amount of time, with confidence in its accuracy and reliability. Physicians often encounter too much information to review in a reasonable period of time and too little specific information that answers a defined question.[6] Patients generally are pleased with their use of the Internet for health searches, but some still find it confusing and frustrating.[14] Interestingly, in focus groups the author conducted with people living with chronic disease, patients also cited a precision issue: finding information of sufficient depth and specificity relative to gender, age, ethnicity and stage of disease (According to Focus Group discussions for NLM/NIH grant on chronic disease, May 2006, Center for Health and Healing, Beth Israel Medical Center, New York).

INTEGRATIVE MEDICINE AND THE PRIMARY CARE PHYSICIAN

Although some primary care physicians may choose to move toward the practice of integrative health care, many recognize the need to become more informed about the efficacy and safety of the therapies their patients may be using. In either case, there are a set of questions that are useful for physicians to answer in order to confidently and capably deal with the practice of medicine in this new environment (**Box 1**).

> **Box 1**
> **Questions concerning integrative health care**
>
> What is the basis and mechanism of action of integrative therapies?
>
> What is the evidence-base for their effectiveness?
>
> How do these therapies compare with standard medical practice in treating various health conditions?
>
> What are the interactions between herbal and dietary supplements and pharmaceuticals?
>
> How effective and safe are integrative approaches for various health conditions?
>
> What are the potential adverse effects?
>
> How do specific herbs and supplements interact with laboratory tests?
>
> How can one identify high-quality herbal medicines and dietary supplements?
>
> What are the training and licensing parameters for each approach?
>
> How can one find trained, certified, or licensed practitioners?
>
> How can one identify reliable online resources and help guide patients to them?

A GUIDE TO INTEGRATIVE MEDICINE ON THE INTERNET

The online resources described have been selected for their usefulness in clinical practice and their adherence to sound principles of credibility and reliability, as outlined at the end of this article. They provide referenced overviews of topics, relevant research, practitioner referral lists, and online education on the integrative approach to health and wellness.

Resources listed by therapeutic modality follow the NIH classification system[15] and have been selected for their clinically relevant content. Because of this specific focus, many sites important to the practice of these approaches are not included, as they primarily address professional practice issues rather than information of use to the primary care physician.

Additional sections cover authoritative online resources geared to the patient, specialized relevant databases, and a short tutorial on Web site evaluation.

LOCATING INFORMATION QUICKLY
Search Engines

Site retrieval by search engines depends on many factors, the least of which may be the authority of the site. Because of this it is important to create the best search possible using the strategies that are available on each search engine. An example on Google is shown in **Box 2**.

Specialized Medical Search Engines

A recent study found a 31% increase in the reliability of information retrieved when using a specialized medical search engine, although this still represents a reliability factor of only 72%.[16] Medical search engines can help one refine a search and focus results. Two such sites are

Medstory (http://www.medstory.com). Developed by experts in artificial intelligence and cognitive science, this site retrieves highly relevant quality content providing targeted information quickly. Categories include procedures, nutrition, complementary medicine, drugs, audio/video formats, and types of information (news stories, clinical trials, research studies).

Box 2
Search strategies for Google

Use the Advanced Search feature to limit to specific domains such as .edu, .gov or .org.

Focus results by putting phrases in quotation marks, a plus sign (+) before a word that must occur in your results and a minus sign (−) before a word you want to exclude. For example, *migraines + relaxation - biofeedback* will retrieve results on relaxation approaches for migraines other than biofeedback.

Type in a health condition (with or without a second search term) and then click on Show Options at the top of the page. Select Reviews from the left menu bar to retrieve generally high-quality reviews on the selected topic. For example, Diabetes Dietary Supplements.

Google Scholar (http://scholar.google.com) covers peer-reviewed papers, theses, books, and scholarly articles. In Advanced Search, retrieval can be limited to Medicine or a specific author or journal. Results are weighted by author, publication, and number of times cited in the scholarly literature.

Healia (http://www.healia.com). This special NIH-funded technology improves search quality by providing other related search words, subcategories (causes, symptoms, diagnosis, and treatment), and filters (gender, age, and ethnicity).

Other key sites are shown in **Box 3**.

EBM Databases

These include

SUM search (University of Texas)—http://sumsearch.uthscsa.edu/. This meta-searcher for evidence-based health information searches several Internet

---

Box 3
Key sites

EBM reviews

Cochrane Library: complementary medicine field (http://www.cochrane.org/reviews/en/topics/22_reviews.html)

Clinical information

Wake Forest University School of Medicine, Program for Holistic & Integrative Medicine (http://www.besthealth.com/Integrated+Medicine)

Online learning/CME

University of Minnesota, The Center for Spirituality & Healing Healthcare Professional Series: Online Modules (http://www.csh.umn.edu/modules/index.html)

Supplement database

Memorial Sloan Kettering Cancer Center: about herbs, botanicals and other products (http://www.mskcc.org/mskcc/html/11570.cfm)

Supplement database, subscription

Natural Medicines Comprehensive Database (http://www.naturaldatabase.com)

Consumer sites

University of Maryland Medical Center (http://www.umm.edu/altmed/)

University of Minnesota, Taking Charge of Your Health (http://takingcharge.csh.umn.edu/)

sources at once: DARE (Database of Reviews of Effects, including Cochrane reviews), PubMed (MEDLINE), guidelines clearinghouses, and more. Results are organized from broadest to narrowest level of information and include review articles, practice guidelines, systematic reviews, and textbooks.

TRIP database (Center for Research Support)—http://www.tripdatabase.com. This collection of hyperlinks to high-quality medical information from EBM sites includes systematic reviews, evidence-based synopses, guidelines, peer-reviewed journals, and "eTextbooks." It is updated monthly.

Cochrane Library: Complementary Medicine Field—http://www.cochrane.org/reviews/en/topics/22_reviews.html. This free version of the Cochrane Library provides EBM abstract reviews on integrative therapies including herbal and dietary supplements, mind–body medicine, manual medicine, and traditional systems of medicine. The site contains hundreds of systematic reviews representing a high level of evidence.

eCAM-Evidence-Based Complementary and Alternative Medicine from Oxford Journals—http://ecam.oxfordjournals.org/. This international, peer-reviewed journal database covers research on integrative medicine and CAM. Articles are available with full text.

Integrative Medicine on Medline

CAM on PubMed (http://www.nlm.nih.gov/nccam/camonpubmed.html) automatically limits searches on PubMed to articles on integrative and complementary medicine. Searches can be limited in Publication Types to meta-analyses or randomized controlled trials.

Clinical Resources on Integrative Approaches

These include

Department of Family Medicine, University of Wisconsin-Madison, Integrative Medicine Program (http://www.fammed.wisc.edu/integrative/modules). Teaching modules and patient handouts on the integrative approach to a variety of health conditions including depression, gastroesophageal reflux disease (GERD), headaches, hypertension, irritable bowel syndrome (IBS), osteoarthritis, and more.

Essential Evidence Plus (http://www.essentialevidenceplus.com/index.cfm). This subscription service provides up-to-date POEMs (Patient-Oriented Evidence that Matters), information based on relevant clinical questions and measurable patient outcomes. The Daily POEMs feature E-mails subscribers the most valid, relevant research that impacts clinical practice.

NCCAM NIH (http://nccam.nih.gov/). This extensive Web site contains information on integrative approaches, consensus reports, and clinical trials. Select Health Information, Diseases and Conditions for reports on integrative approaches to certain diseases and research to date. This site provides a useful introduction to the field.

University of Texas MD Anderson Cancer Center Complementary/Integrative Medicine Education Resources (http://www.mdanderson.org/departments/CIMER/). Select Therapies for scientific reviews on systems of medicine (Chinese medicine, Ayurveda, homeopathy), herbal medicine, nutritional therapies, manual medicine, energy therapies, mind–body approaches, and cancer. These reviews vary in depth and scope.

Wake Forest University School of Medicine, Program for Holistic & Integrative Medicine (http://www.besthealth.com/Integrated+Medicine). Provides comprehensive information on treating health conditions through a combination of conventional medical treatments and integrative approaches including nutrition, herbal medicine, homeopathy, acupuncture, and mind–body medicine.

Online Learning in Integrative Medicine: Tutorials, CME Courses, Web Casts and Videos

Online learning opportunities include

Bastyr University (http://www.bastyr.edu/library/resources/researchguide/cammedline.asp). This site provides practical searching guides to integrative research on PubMed and evidence-based resources on acupuncture, botanicals, and naturopathic medicine. Access is free.

CamPODS by CAM UME (Complementary and Alternative Medicine Issues in Undergraduate Medical Education) (http://www.caminume.ca/drr/campods.html). These peer-reviewed summaries developed primarily for medical school instructors include the foundation of CAM, CAM in clinical practice, and particular CAM therapies. Access is free.

NCCAM, Online Continuing Education Series (http://nccam.nih.gov/videolectures/index.htm). These short CME/continuing education modules cover herbs and dietary supplements, mind–body medicine, acupuncture, manual therapies, aging, and more. Each includes a video lecture, question-and-answer transcript, optional online test, resource links, and certificate of completion. A maximum of 10 CME Category I credits and 12 CE contact hours will be awarded. Access is free.

University of Minnesota: The Center for Spirituality & Healing Healthcare Professional Series: Online Modules (http://www.csh.umn.edu/modules/index.html). This well-designed online program offers 16 modules on topics in the field of integrative medicine. Each module takes from 1 to 3.5 hours to complete. The learning objectives support the following competencies: Accreditation Council for Graduate Medical Education (ACGME) for Medical education, AACN for Nursing education, and AACP for Pharmacy education. Access is free.

National Cancer Institute (NCI): Office of Cancer Complementary and Alternative Medicine (OCCAM) Best Case Series Program (http://www.cancer.gov/cam/bestcase_intro.html). OCCAM coordinates the NCI's research program in CAM. Since 1991, the NCI has had a scientifically rigorous Best Case Series Program that provides an independent review of medical records and medical imaging from patients treated with therapies outside of conventional medicine. Access is free.

University of Arizona College of Medicine Program in Integrative Medicine Online Education Courses (http://integrativemedicine.arizona.edu/education/online_courses.html). Web-based courses on topics in integrative medicine include online material, required and recommended reading, virtual patients, and a three-CD set of interviews. Series includes nutrition and health, botanical medicine, and whole systems of medicine. Access is fee-based. CME credit is available.

University of North Carolina at Chapel Hill, Program on Integrative Medicine Monographs on Integrative Medicine: Educational Resources for Health Professionals (http://pim.med.unc.edu/Monographs.html). These monographs are part of a series of publications entitled *The Convergence of Complementary, Alternative*

& *Conventional Health Care* developed as an educational resource for health professionals. PDF versions of each monograph can be downloaded for free.

Integrative Therapies and Systems of Medicine

The following resources provide information on specific therapeutic approaches that are increasingly becoming a part of integrative health care. Sites were selected for their relevance to clinical issues, particularly research in the field and practitioner locators.

Whole medical systems

Acupuncture and East Asian Medicine The resources include

Acubriefs (http://www.acubriefs.com). Sponsored by the Medical Acupuncture Research Foundation, this free, easy to search database contains over 16,000 citations on acupuncture, many with online links to PubMed.

Tufts University: The Evidence-Based Complementary and Alternative Medicine Program–East Asian Medicine (EAM) (http://www.tufts.edu/med/ebcam/). Focuses on Chinese herbal medicine, acupuncture, and exercises such as Tai Chi and Qigong. Research evidence is detailed, and the appropriateness of referral to a practitioner is evaluated. EAM interventions for cardiovascular health, smoking cessation, and hypertension are reviewed in depth.

Acupuncture.com (http://www.acupuncture.com). This site provides a referral database by geographic area.

Ayurveda The resources include

The Ayurveda Institute (http://www.ayurveda.com/). The Online Resource section provides a good overview of the Ayurvedic approach to health; specific information on food, nutrition, and cleansing procedures; and the basic elements of Ayurveda.

National Center for Complementary and Alternative Medicine, NIH (http://nccam.nih.gov/health/ayurveda/). This site provides a good overview of Ayurveda's use in the United States, underlying concepts, treatments, practitioner training and certification, Ayurvedic herbs, and NCCAM-funded research.

Homeopathy The resources include

National Center for Homeopathy (http://homeopathic.org/). This site provides a wide variety of information including a practitioner database and a research section covering meta-analyses and peer-reviewed articles.

Hom-Inform British Homeopathic Library at Glasgow Homeopathic Hospital (http://www.hom-inform.org/). This database contains approximately 20,000 references dating back to 1911. Searching is free; copies of articles can be ordered.

British Homeopathic Association and Homeopathic Trust (http://www.trusthomeopathy.org). The Research section provides an introduction to the kinds of evidence that exist for homeopathy and the range of conditions where positive findings have been reported in at least one systematic review, randomized controlled trial or nonrandomized study.

Naturopathy The resources include

Bastyr Center for Natural Health, Bastyr University (http://www.bastyrcenter.org/). The Health Conditions section provides an overview and links to relevant and current research articles on natural approaches to each health condition.

American Association of Naturopathic Medical Colleges (http://www.aanmc.org/). This site provides a good overview of the naturopathic profession in North America.

American Association of Naturopathic Physicians (http://www.naturopathic.org). This site provides a national directory of practitioners.

Heart Spring (http://www.heartspring.net/).

Mind–body medicine

Mindfulness and meditation The resources include

NCCAM, NIH (http://nccam.nih.gov/health/whatiscam/overview.htm). Select Mind–Body Interventions for a referenced overview of mind-body therapies and their specific applications.

Benson-Henry Institute for Mind–Body Medicine (http://www.mbmi.org/home/). The Institute is a world leader in the study, training, and clinical practice of mind—body medicine. Under Mind/Body Basics, the site covers information on stress, the components of mind–body medicine, and strategies for managing stress.

University of Wisconsin, Department of Family Medicine (http://www.fammed.wisc.edu/integrative/modules/meditation). This site provides information for clinicians and patients on clinical benefits, types of meditation, suggested Web sites, and more.

Biofeedback/Neurofeedback The resources include

Association for Applied Psychophysiology and Biofeedback (http://www.aapb.org/). Under Provider's Information, a list of health problems treatable with biofeedback or neurofeedback therapy includes a summary of supporting evidence and efficacy rating on a scale of 1 to 5. The News and Current Research sections provide an up-to-date list of research articles linked to PubMed.

Biofeedback Certification Institute of America (BCIA) (http://www.bcia.org). BCIA certification is a standard in the field. The site maintains a searchable international locator of practitioners and their specific certification.

International Society for Neurofeedback and Research (http://www.isnr.org/). Neurofeedback is a form of biofeedback that focuses on the central nervous system and the brain. Under Comprehensive Neurofeedback Bibliography, this site maintains an up-to-date collection of research studies on neurofeedback for 45 health conditions linked to PubMed.

Guided imagery The resources include

Academy for Guided Imagery (http://www.academyforguidedimagery.com/). Under Research Findings, research reviews are posted on the use of guided imagery for various medical conditions, psychological issues, pediatric health conditions, and medical procedures.

Hypnotherapy The resources include

American Society of Clinical Hypnosis (ASCH) (http://www.asch.net/). ASCH is the largest US organization for health care professionals using clinical hypnosis. The site provides background information on its medical uses and a searchable member referral database by state.

Biologically based practices

Herbs/Supplements The resources include

University of Maryland Herbal Database (http://www.umm.edu/altmed/index.htm). This site has evidence-based information covering overview, indications, pediatric and adult dosage, precautions, interactions, references, and more. Links to conditions for which herbs are used, herbs with similar uses, drugs that interact, and herbs with similar warnings.

Memorial Sloan Kettering Cancer Center: About Herbs, Botanicals and Other Products (http://www.mskcc.org/mskcc/html/11570.cfm). This site contains full-text evidence-based information with citations linked to PubMed on an extensive list of herbs, vitamins, and supplements. A clinical summary for each agent is provided as well as details about plant constituents, adverse effects, herb–drug interactions, laboratory interactions, and potential benefits or problems.

IBIDS (The International Bibliographic Information on Dietary Supplements database) (http://ods.od.nih.gov/databases/ibids.html). This site covers the worldwide scientific literature on vitamins, minerals, and botanic supplements from 1986 to the present. The database can be searched in two ways: the complete database or peer-reviewed citations only.

IBIDS Clinical (http://ibids.nal.usda.gov/clinical/). This pilot version of IBIDS Clinical is geared to clinical practice and research. Records on important supplements list meta-analyses, systematic reviews, practice guidelines, consensus statements, and position papers from 1994 to the present. The site is in continuous development and provides a very concise way to locate high-quality information.

Subscription databases
These include

Natural Medicines Comprehensive Database (http://www.naturaldatabase.com). This site contains thorough detailed monographs covering almost every herb and supplement. It provides reliable, clinically relevant, and evidence-based full-text information arranged to answer clinicians' questions on uses, interactions, and efficacy. The site was developed by pharmacists for health professionals.

Natural Standard (http://www.naturalstandard.com). Developed by clinicians and researchers from over 100 academic institutions, this EBM resource covers herbs, supplements, food, integrative therapies, and health conditions. It provides extensive, referenced, evaluated, and graded scientific information in three levels: professional monograph, bottom-line monograph, and flash-card quick reference summary or patient handout. A Comparative Effectiveness database ranks appropriate therapies per disease by level of evidence.

Nutrition The resources include

Harvard School of Public Health: The Nutrition Source (http://www.hsph.harvard.edu/nutritionsource/). This site provides timely information on diet and nutrition for clinicians and consumers. It offers a healthy eating pyramid, summarizing the most up-to-date dietary information in an easy-to-use format.

Tufts University: The Evidence-Based Complementary and Alternative Medicine Program–Nutrition (http://www.tufts.edu/med/ebcam/nutrition/index.html). This site includes evidence-based information on supplements, vitamins, probiotics, and antioxidants. Additionally it has reviews of nutritional approaches for health conditions including cardiovascular disease, type 2 diabetes, hypertension, HIV and weight loss as well as clinical resources including patient handouts, PowerPoint presentations, and more.

Oldways Preservation and Exchange Trust (http://www.oldwayspt.org/). This site provides culturally sensitive, evidence-based guides for healthy eating through Asian, Latin, Mediterranean, and vegetarian pyramids.

Manual and body-based practices

Osteopathy The sites include

American Osteopathic Association (AOA) (http://www.am-osteo-assn.org). This site provides an online physician locator for all AOA doctors trained in osteopathic manipulative treatments (OMT).

Journal of the American Osteopathic Association (JAOA) (http://www.jaoa.org/). This is an easy-to-use searchable database of the osteopathic literature published in JAOA.

The Cranial Academy (http://www.cranialacademy.com/researchCLINICAL.html). This site covers the research on cranial osteopathy for health conditions such as otitis media, pregnancy, and neurologic, dental, and learning problems.

Chiropractic The resources include

American Chiropractic Association (http://www.amerchiro.org/). Under Patients, find an online chiropractor locator.

Chiropractic Education and Research (http://www.fcer.org/). DCConsult is a clinician/patient research information resource. One can search by keyword, journal, or author on the Medline database for scientific evidence relevant to a patient's condition and treatment.

Massage The resources include

American Massage Therapy Association (http://www.amtamassage.org/). A massage therapy research database provides the latest information on the efficacy of massage and other specific techniques. This site also has a massage therapist locator by state.

Touch Research Institute, University of Miami (TRI) (http://www6.miami.edu/touch-research/). TRI is the first academic center devoted solely to the study of touch and its clinical applications, conducting over 100 studies across all age groups. A team of researchers provides research abstracts for massage, tai chi, and yoga.

Movement therapies: yoga, tai chi, qigong Available resources include

Agency for Healthcare Research and Quality (AHRQ): Meditation Practices for Health: State of the Research, June 2007 (http://www.ahrq.gov/downloads/pub/evidence/pdf/meditation/medit.pdf). This site covers the research on mindfulness and mantra meditation, yoga, tai chi, and qi gong published in the medical and psychological literature.

American Tai Chi Association Digital Library (http://www.americantaichi.net/). Select the Digital library for a quick and easy way to search Medline for articles on tai chi for health conditions including arthritis, balance issues, cardiovascular diseases, musculoskeletal disorders, and many more.

QiGong Institute (http://www.qigonginstitute.org). This site provides access to full text articles on Qigong from the journal literature and a practitioner locator by state and country. The QiGong Database contains over 4000 abstracts available on a pay-per-abstract basis.

Energy medicine: reiki and therapeutic touch

Therapeutic touch The resources include

Nurse-Healers Professional Association (http://www.therapeutic-touch.org/). The official organization for Therapeutic Touch, the Web site provides information on its practice and a geographic listing of teachers.

Healing Touch International (http://www.healingtouchinternational.org/). The professional nonprofit organization for Healing Touch, the site has a practitioner and instructor locator and an annotated list of healing touch research in 16 categories including cancer, cardiovascular, stress, the elderly, and pain.

CamLine   (http://www.camline.ca/camtherapies/camtp.php?camtplistingID=2). This site provides an evidence-based review on therapeutic touch covering efficacy, adverse effects, scope of practice, education, and regulation.

Reiki The resources include

International Association of Reiki Professionals (http://www.reiki.org). This site provides general information on Reiki, a Reiki practitioner and teacher locator, and a database of Reiki articles.

Patient Sites

These include

Aetna InteliHealth (http://www.intelihealth.com/). Aetna InteliHealth provides disease and treatment overviews, including evidence-based information on integrative approaches to common health conditions.

Bastyr Center for Natural Health, Bastyr University (http://bastyrcenter.org/content/category/3/130/186/). This site provides a natural therapies approach to health conditions.

CAM, MedlinePlus (http://www.nlm.nih.gov/medlineplus/complementaryandalternativemedicine.html). This site has consumer health links from the NLM. It is a good jumping off point.

Center for Health and Healing, Beth Israel Medical Center (http://www.health andhealingny.org). Developed by the author, the site provides overviews, research, and resources on 30 integrative approaches and traditional medicines and a Health A to Z section annotating high-quality research on 66 health conditions. Special multimedia modules present the integrative approach to chronic pain, depression, heart disease, diabetes, and IBS.

CARE (Complementary and Alternative Research and Education Program), University of Alberta (http://www.care.ualberta.ca/resources.htm). This site has clinical summaries on common pediatric complaints including asthma, eczema, common cold, diarrhea, infantile colic, and ear infection. The therapy is rated by safety and effectiveness.

ConsumerLab (http://www.consumerlab.com). This site provides independent test results on product quality of common brands of vitamins, minerals, and dietary supplements. It also has referenced information on health conditions, supplements, functional foods, drug interactions, and homeopathy. Complete information is available for a small yearly fee, which pays for the research done by the site.

Health Journeys (http://www.healthjourneys.com/). Developed by a pioneer in the field of imagery and health, the site provides research information, a collection of high-quality resources on wellness, health disorders, chronic illness, practice tips, and a discussion forum.

MedlinePlus Herbs and Supplements (http://www.nlm.nih.gov/medlineplus/druginfo/herb_All.html). This site has high-quality herbal monographs prepared by the Natural Standard Research Collaboration with use rated by scientific evidence, dosing information, interactions, and more.

NIH Senior Health: CAM (http://nihseniorhealth.gov/). This site describes NIH-funded research on integrative approaches to diseases that affect older adults including heart disease, cancer, arthritis, and Alzheimer's disease.

Taking Charge of Your Health, Center for Health and Spirituality, University of Minnesota (http://takingcharge.csh.umn.edu). This is an innovative, high-quality Web site for consumers on the integrative approach to health, getting the most from the current health care system, and creating a healthy lifestyle.

The New Medicine (http://thenewmedicine.org/). This site focuses on prevention strategies and engaging people in their health care. An A-to-Z section of health conditions covers integrative approaches that have been shown to be beneficial. My Health Planner helps patients create and track their own plan for more balanced health and wellbeing.

University of Maryland Medical Center (http://www.umm.edu/altmed/). This an authoritative and informative introduction to the most common integrative approaches, from acupuncture to yoga.

World's Healthiest Foods (George Mateljan Foundation, http://www.whfoods.org/). This nonprofit foundation publicizes scientific information about the benefits of healthy eating. Under Getting Started, the sections on eating healthy and cooking healthy contain a wealth of referenced information.

Web Site Evaluation Guidelines

Without consistent editorial systems or peer review, the quality of information on the Internet varies widely. The following evaluation criteria culled by the author from

---

Box 4
Web site evaluation: how to assess credibility

Who wrote or produced the site?

> A university or medical center, a government agency, a library, a consumer group, a commercial sponsor or an individual? Look for well-known and respected sources.

Is the information current?

> Medical knowledge is evolving constantly, so it is important that information is current. The site should note the date when specific information was written, and the date of the site's update should be posted. Be sure to look for these dates.

What is the source of the information?

> The site should give the names of the authors who wrote the content and the names of journals or books where the content appeared.

Are the people who wrote the content experts in their field?

> The site should tell the credentials of the authors so one can evaluate if their education and experience is appropriate for the information they are giving.

Does the site talk about the benefits and risks of treatments, how a treatment works, or what other treatments might also work?

> The site should provide you with balanced information. If the site claims a treatment is a cure or works all the time, that should be a red flag: it's important to know on what evidence that statement is based.

Look for a rating system

> An HONCode or URAC label appearing on the site is like a Good Housekeeping Seal of Approval. It tells you that certain criteria have been met regarding the quality and reliability of the health information on that site.

many authoritative sources over the years will help in selecting reliable online resources. The most important factor to assess is the credibility of the site. Various criteria can help in this process.

Publisher (who runs, pays for and publishes the site?)

Look for well-known and respected sources such as universities, research centers, libraries, hospitals, journals, government agencies, and professional organizations. Consumer advocacy groups, voluntary health-related organizations, and provider organizations also can provide credible information.

Web sites published by commercial sponsors and professional and lay individuals may seem like biased sources, but following the evaluative criteria listed here will help distinguish those that are reliable.

Authority (expertise in the field)

Look for clearly identified authorship or source, including authors' educational backgrounds, credentials, affiliations, publications, and experience.

All references to other publications should be identified with the correct and full bibliographic citation.

Editorial practices, reviewers, advisory board members, or consultants should be identified.

Trustworthiness (assessment of bias)

The site should include disclosure of its mission, purpose, standards for posting information, potential conflicts of interest, and use of information gathered about users.

Appropriate disclaimers that address a site's limitations and scope should be posted.

The opportunity for interactivity through E-mail should be available.

Content quality

Medical sites should be updated regularly and frequently, with the most recent update or review date posted.

While information accuracy can be difficult to evaluate, the substance and depth of content may help to determine this. Is the coverage basic or comprehensive? Is the presentation objective and balanced?

Content should be understandable relative to the site's intended users.

Links should be accurate, current, credible, and relevant. The policy for choosing links should be noted. Are there specific criteria? Is there a charge to link?

Links between sites should match the original site's audience, allow free movement between sites, and be selective.

Design quality

Site organization and technology should help to locate information quickly and easily.

Site aesthetics including color, lack of clutter, and legibility of text should contribute to comfort and ease of use.

Various text, audio, and video formats allow for differences in the ways users learn.

Rating system

An HONCode or URAC label indicates certain criteria have been met relative to the authority and safety of health information. Not all good sites have it, but it is a start.

Box 4 shows a simplified version of these evaluation criteria that providers can share with their patients. It addresses the basic issues affecting site authority and reliability.

Table 1
Types of Web sites

Type of Site	URL	Description
Search engines	http://www.google.com	General search engine
	http://www.scholar.google.com	General search engine
	http://www.medstory.com	Medical search engine
	http://www.healia.com	Medical search engine
Evidence-based medicine (EBM)	http://www.cochrane.org/reviews/en/topics/22_reviews.html	EBM resources and research reviews
	http://sumsearch.uthscsa.edu/	EBM resources and research reviews
	http://www.tripdatabase.com	EBM resources and research reviews
	http://ecam.oxfordjournals.org/	EBM resources and research reviews
PubMed/CAM	http://www.nlm.nih.gov/nccam/camonpubmed.html	Medline searching focused on CAM
Integrative medicine clinical resources	http://www.fammed.wisc.edu/integrative/modules	Teaching modules, patient handouts
	http://www.essentialevidenceplus.com/index.cfm	Clinical research-based information
	http://www.besthealth.com/Integrated+Medicine	Clinical information
	http://nccam.nih.gov/	Good introduction to the field
	http://www.mdanderson.org/departments/CIMER/	Scientific reviews on therapeutic approaches
Online tutorials, CME courses, webcasts and videos	http://www.caminume.ca/drr/campods.html	Peer-reviewed summaries
	http://www.csh.umn.edu/modules/index.html	Online modules on CAM (CME/CE)
	http://www.cancer.gov/cam/bestcase_intro.html	Best case series program
	http://integrativemedicine.arizona.edu/education/online_courses/	Online course on nutrition/herbs, systems of medicine (CME)
	http://pim.med.unc.edu/Monographs.html	Online monographs on integrative topics
	http://nccam.nih.gov/videolectures/index.htm	Video lectures (CME/CE)
	http://www.bastyr.edu/library/resources/researchguide/cammedline.asp	Search guides and resources

(continued on next page)

Table 1
(*continued*)

Type of Site	URL	Description
Systems of medicine	Acupuncture and East Asian medicine	
	http://www.acubriefs.com	Research database
	http://www.tufts.edu/med/ebcam/	Clinical information
	http://www.acupuncture.com	Practitioner referral database
	Ayurveda	
	http://www.ayurveda.com/	Overview
	http://nccam.nih.gov/health/ayurveda/	Overview
	Homeopathy	
	http://homeopathic.org/	Research reviews, referral database
	http://www.hom-inform.org/	Research database
	http://www.trusthomeopathy.org	Clinical information
	Naturopathy	
	http://www.bastyrcenter.org/	Clinical information
	http://www.aanmc.org/	Overview
	http://www.naturopathic.org	Practitioner referral database
Mind–body medicine	Mindfulness and meditation	
	http://nccam.nih.gov/health/whatiscam/overview.htm	Overview and clinical applications
	http://www.mbmi.org/home/	Overview
	http://www.fammed.wisc.edu/integrative/ modules/meditation	Clinical information
	Biofeedback/neurofeedback	
	http://www.aapb.org/	Clinical information
	http://www.bcia.org	Practitioner locator
	http://www.isnr.org/	Research and clinical information
	Guided imagery	
	http://www.academyforguidedimagery.com/	Research and clinical information
	Hypnotherapy	
	http://www.asch.net/	Overview and referral database

Biologically based medicine	**Herbs/supplements**	
	http://www.umm.edu/altmed/index.htm	Clinical herbal monographs
	http://www.mskcc.org/mskcc/html/11570.cfm	Clinical herbal monographs
	http://ods.od.nih.gov/databases/ibids.html	Research database
	http://ibids.nal.usda.gov/clinical/	Research database for clinical practice
	Subscription databases	
	http://www.naturaldatabase.com	Herbal/supplement monographs
	http://www.naturalstandard.com	Herbal/supplement monographs
	Nutrition	
	http://www.hsph.harvard.edu/nutritionsource/	Clinical information
	http://www.tufts.edu/med/ebcam/nutrition/index.html	Clinical information
	http://www.oldwayspt.org/	Patient education
Manual and body-based practices	**Osteopathy**	
	http://www.am-osteo-assn.org	Physician locator
	http://www.jaoa.org/	Research database
	http://www.cranialacademy.com/researchCLINICAL.html	Research and clinical information
	Chiropractic	
	http://www.amerchiro.org/	Practitioner locator
	http://www.fcer.org/	Research database
	Massage	
	http://www.amtamassage.org/	Research database, practitioner locator
	http://www6.miami.edu/touch-research/	Research
	Movement therapies (Yoga, Tai Chi, Qigong)	
	http://www.ahrq.gov/downloads/pub/evidence/pdf/meditation/medit.pdf	Research review
	http://www.americantaichi.net/	Database search
	http://www.qigonginstitute.org	Research and practitioner locator

(continued on next page)

Table 1
(continued)

Type of Site	URL	Description
Energy medicine: Reiki and therapeutic touch	Therapeutic touch	
	http://www.therapeutic-touch.org/	Overview and teacher locator
	http://www.healingtouchinternational.org	Research and practitioner locator
	http://www.camline.ca/camtherapies/camtp.php?camtplistingID=2	Evidence-based overview
	Reiki	
	http://www.reiki.org	Overview and teacher locator
Patient sites	http://www.intelihealth.com/	Treatment overviews
	http://bastyrcenter.org/content/category/3/130/186/	Natural therapies A to Z
	http://www.nlm.nih.gov/medlineplus/complementaryandalternativemedicine.html	Consumer health links from NIH
	http://www.umm.edu/altmed/	Overview from acupuncture to yoga
	http://www.healthandhealingny.org	Overview, research and resources
	http://www.consumerlab.com	Evaluations of herbs/dietary supplements
	http://www.healthjourneys.com	High-quality mind–body resources
	http://www.nlm.nih.gov/medlineplus/druginfo/herb_All.html	Authoritative herbal monographs
	http://nihseniorhealth.gov/	Integrative approach for older adults
	http://takingcharge.csh.umn.edu	Creating a healthy lifestyle
	http://thenewmedicine.org/	Prevention strategies/health planner
	http://www.whfoods.org/	Eating healthy and cooking healthy

SUMMARY

As health care faces profound changes in this country, interest in the contribution of an integrative approach that engages the full range of physical, psychological, social, preventive, and therapeutic strategies to health and disease has grown steadily. With this, the depth, reliability, and accessibility of information on integrative approaches should continue to evolve and provide physicians and consumers with useful and relevant online resources to meet their information needs. The sites selected in this article (**Table 1**) will enable providers to rapidly locate targeted information on integrative approaches and to help build collaborative relationships with patients through educating them about high-quality online resources.

REFERENCES

1. Wilson P. How to find the good and avoid the bad or ugly: a short guide to tools for rating quality of health information on the Internet. BMJ 2002;324(7337): 598–602.
2. Greenberg L, D'andrea G, Lorence D. Setting the public agenda for online health search: a white paper and action agenda. J Med Internet Res 2004; 6(2):e18.
3. Merrell RC, Cone SW, Rafiq A. The authority and utility of Internet information. Stud Health Technol Inform 2008;131:265–72.
4. Adams SA, de Bont AA. More than just a mouse click: research into work practices behind the assignment of medical trust marks on the World Wide Web. Int J Med Inf 2007;76(Suppl 1):S14–20.
5. Casebeer L, Bennett N, Kristofco R, et al. Physicians Internet medical information seeking and on-line continuing education use patterns. J Contin Educ Health Prof 2002;22(1):33–42.
6. Bennett NL, Casebeer LL, Kristofco RE, et al. Physicians' Internet information-seeking behaviors. J Contin Educ Health Prof 2004;24(1):31–8.
7. Owen DJ, Fang ML. Information-seeking behavior in complementary and alternative medicine (CAM): an online survey of faculty at a health sciences campus. J Med Libr Assoc 2003;91(3):311–21.
8. Fox S. Online health search 2006. Washington, DC: Pew Internet & American Life Project; 2006. Pew Internet Project reports: health. Available at: http://www.pewin ternet.org/pdfs/PIP_Online_Health_2006.pdf. Accessed January 27, 2009.
9. McMullan M. Patients using the Internet to obtain health information: how this affects the patient–health professional relationship. Patient Educ Couns 2006; 63:24–8.
10. Rainie L. Testimony to the White House Commission on complementary and alternative medicine policy. Pew Internet & American Life Project. Available at: http:// www.pewinternet.org/ppt/Rainie_Testimony_Alt_Med.pdf. Accessed January 27, 2009.
11. Barnes PM, Bloom B, Nahin RL. Complementary and alternative medicine use among adults and children: United States, 2007. National health statistics reports; No. 12. Hyattsville (MD): National Center for Health Statistics; 2008. Available at: http://www.cdc.gov/nchs/data/nhsr/nhsr012.pdf. Accessed February 18, 2009.
12. Sillence E, Briggs P, Fishwick L. Noting changes in online health: the rise of less regulated Web sites. Health Info Internet 2007;57:6–8.
13. Coulter A, Entwistle V, Gilbert D. Sharing decisions with patients: is the information good enough? BMJ 1999;318:318–22.

14. Pew Internet & American life project tracking surveys (March 2000–May 2008). Available at: http://www.pewinternet.org/trends/Internet_Activities_7.22.08.htm. Accessed February 18, 2009.

15. National Center for Complementary and Alternative Medicine. What is CAM? Available at: http://nccam.nih.gov/health/whatiscam/overview.htm. Accessed May 11, 2009.

16. Gaudinat A, Ruch P, Joubert M, et al. Health search engine with e-document analysis for reliable search results. Int J Med Inf 2006;75(1):73–85.

Index

Note: Page numbers of article titles are in **boldface** type.

Prim Care Clin Office Pract 37 (2010) 201–211
doi:10.1016/S0095-4543(10)00009-6
0095-4543/10/$ – see front matter © 2010 Elsevier Inc. All rights reserved.

primarycare.theclinics.com

Moving?

Make sure your subscription moves with you!

To notify us of your new address, find your **Clinics Account Number** (located on your mailing label above your name), and contact customer service at:

Email: journalscustomerservice-usa@elsevier.com

800-654-2452 (subscribers in the U.S. & Canada)
314-447-8871 (subscribers outside of the U.S. & Canada)

Fax number: 314-447-8029

Elsevier Health Sciences Division
Subscription Customer Service
3251 Riverport Lane
Maryland Heights, MO 63043

*To ensure uninterrupted delivery of your subscription, please notify us at least 4 weeks in advance of move.

Printed and bound by CPI Group (UK) Ltd, Croydon, CR0 4YY

03/10/2024

01040453-0004